QZ
200

LIVING
WITH
CANCER

LIVING WITH CANCER

Mary Moster

HODDER AND STOUGHTON
LONDON SYDNEY AUCKLAND TORONTO

All Scripture quotations are taken from the King James Version, unless otherwise noted.

Scripture quotations from the New American Standard Bible, © 1960, 1962, 1963, 1968, 1971, 1973, and 1975 by the Lockman Foundation, are used by permission.

British Library Cataloguing in Publication Data
Moster, Mary
  Living with cancer.—2nd ed.—(Hodder
Christian paperbacks).
  1. Cancer—Religious aspects—Christianity
  I. Title
  248.8'6   BT732

ISBN 0-340-42222-X

Hodder and Stoughton Editorial Office: 47 Bedford Square, London WC1B 3DP

To Steve

for his confidence and encouragement

CONTENTS

FOREWORD

By Dr Roger Hurding

Cancer, for the majority of people, is the most feared disease. Though AIDS is beginning to compete for this doubtful honour, it is the possibility of cancer that haunts so many patients as they seek medical advice on their puzzling symptoms. I can readily recall, in my years as a principal in General Practice, the frequency of the pressing question, 'Is it cancer, doctor?'

Why is cancer so feared? There are many reasons but it is primarily because it is seen as *common*, *painful* and *fatal*.

Overall, the incidence of malignant disease *is* high in the so-called 'developed' countries—not least because of the increasingly large population of the elderly. Something like one in three people will contract cancer during their lifetime and, therefore, the number affected, including relatives and friends of the afflicted, is vast.

Though the public readily associates suffering from cancer with a great deal of pain, the link is not inevitable. In fact, the early stages of this illness are usually pain-free. In advanced disease, pain is preventable. Dr Cicely Saunders, the founder of the Hospice Movement, has pointed out that half those with cancer experience little or no discomfort, one in ten have mild pain and the remainder can be kept comfortable by the use of drugs (see p.141).

Just as cancer is not inevitably painful so it is not invariably fatal. Though there is no doubt that cancer is a common cause of death (up to one in four in the United Kingdom), there are certain forms and stages of malignancy which can be readily treated, and even cured, by surgical and medical means. For example: skin cancers are often identified early and are thus completely removable; Hodgkin's disease and testicular cancers frequently respond well to chemotherapy; and tumours of the mouth and larynx can be cleared up completely by radiation. Medical progress is leading to further success in the treatment of cancer. Since 1980, for instance, the death rate from childhood leukaemia has dropped by nearly sixty per cent. It has to be said, too, that many cancers (particularly those relating to smoking, heavy drinking of alcohol, exposure to toxic chemicals and excessive sunlight, and sexual promiscuity) are preventable.

In the light of these understandable fears of not only developing cancer but of having to face pain and death itself from the spread of malignancy, what is needed is a book that is both realistic and encouraging. *Living with Cancer* is just such a book. Mary Moster, the author and a journalist, had, like so many of us, close relatives who contracted cancer. Her mother is a cancer sufferer, a grandmother died of cancer of the breast and her sister-in-law, Jan, developed a terminal brain tumour within two years of marriage.

It was through the latter's illness that Mary Moster met Nell Collins, a Christian nurse who had herself known the fear and panic of being faced with her own cancer. Having been on the receiving end of surgery and chemotherapy, Nell became, in time, a 'full-time missionary to cancer patients'. She is one of those 'missionaries of comfort' who take Paul's words in 2 Corinthians 1:3,4 very seriously indeed:

> Praise be to the God and Father of our Lord Jesus Christ, the Father of compassion and the God of all comfort, who comforts us in all our troubles, so that we can comfort those in any trouble with the comfort we ourselves have received from God [NIV].

Through her direct experience of Jan's death under the age of twenty-five and through her friendship with Nell Collins, Mary Moster has written a book which is brimful with good sense and godly wisdom, amply illustrated with stories of Nell's patients and others. Everyday questions of living with cancer are tackled with honesty: How can I cope with my changed 'body-image' after surgery? What side-effects might I have following chemotherapy? How can we cope as a family, knowing our loved one is dying? How should we treat our child now we know he has cancer? Should we tell his brother and sister? Where can I get the special equipment my ill wife needs? How can we get financial help now my husband has cancer? At what stage might the local hospice be involved? The book is a mine of practical information, including facts and figures about the various forms of cancer and a range of useful addresses.

Throughout *Living with Cancer* there is a blend of home truths and heavenly perspectives. In fact, the 'heavenly perspectives' are as down-to-earth as the 'home truths' in the practical godliness of Nell Collins. This 'full-time missionary to cancer patients' offers her charges a friendship which is prepared to listen and advise in any area of their need. At times, this level of caring is able to be quite open about the Christ who is able 'to sympathise with our weaknesses' (Heb. 4:15 [NIV]). In one instance, Douglas Evans, whose earthly hopes had been shattered through progressive illness, found, in Nell's sensitive response to his questions, a new hope through his relationship with the 'blessed Controller of all things' (p.74).

And yet, Mary Moster offers no easy answers. She does not sidestep the seemingly unanswerable questions. Why me, God? Why, as one woman asked, should I, aged thirty-two and with a boy of six, have cancer of the breast? Is God always good? What about miracles? Why does God heal some and not others? How can God help me cope with death and dying? What lies beyond the grave?

It is in the face of these imponderables that Christian hope has a special place. The New Testament often makes the link between hope and endurance. It is as patient, friends and family open their lives to Christ that they are given strength to persevere. The body may be subject to wasting and weakness but with 'Christ in you, the hope of glory' (Col. 1:27 [NIV]) ultimate victory is assured. As one Christian sixteen year old, after four years battling with a brain tumour, wrote:

> Cancer is cruel, crippling and callous, but even if it cannot always be cured, it can be *conquered*.[1]

Perhaps, much as in any other situation in life, living with cancer can be, in spite of all the discouragements and setbacks, a living out of God's all-sufficiency. The path is never easy, but Christ can be the loving companion on the way. Mary Moster tells how Nell Collins, following her own renewed commitment to the Lord, put it like this:

> Then there was peace in the midst of turmoil, joy in the face of sorrow, hopelessness turned to hope, and fear turned to trust (p.3).

Roger F Hurding

ACKNOWLEDGMENTS

Many people have participated in this effort by giving generously of their time and understanding. I would like to thank each one of them by name, but, of course, that is impossible. To all of the cancer patients, the families, various medical people, and counsellors who helped make this book possible I give my heartfelt thanks.

Pastors Wendell T. Heller and Donald J. Kouwe have given greatly appreciated help and guidance. Pastor Charles E. Perry, Jr, has devoted many hours to reading and checking the manuscript, and I thank him for his important contributions.

Peter Scott, MD, a radiologist at St Vincent's Hospital in Indianapolis, gave of his time to check the manuscript from the medical point of view. Arthur Provisor, MD, assistant professor of paediatrics in the division of haematology/oncology at James Whitcomb Riley Hospital for Children in Indianapolis was extremely helpful, as was Pam Flummer-felt, RN, in giving me counsel on the problems of childhood cancer.

I also thank Rene Mastrovito, MD, of the staff of Memorial Sloan-Kettering Cancer Center in New York for his permission to use a number of quotations from the Center's *Clinical Bulletin*.

I appreciate the information made available through the American Cancer Society as well as material from the Public Health Service, National Institutes of Health, and the United States Department of Health, Education, and Welfare.

The British edition was made possible through the helpfulness of many British cancer charities, and in particular I would like to thank BACUP (British Association of Cancer United Patients). Special thanks also go to Penelope Brock, MD, Leukaemia Research Fellow at Great Ormond Street Hospital for Sick Children, for giving so generously of her time.

Susie Logston and Beverly Moore helped by reading over the manuscript, and I thank Sally Tanselle for her editorial counsel.

Several wonderful Bible teachers have indirectly participated in this book by patiently, lovingly, and consistently teaching what God says in his Word. I particularly thank Dick and Bev Anthony, Ralph and Ann Walls, Chris Harrold, Cindy Zeigler, Jim Gamble, and Ed Runyan. I also thank my parents, Mr and Mrs Tom Mattox, and Mr and Mrs Ernie Copple for their love and concern.

Most especially, I want to thank Nell Collins for pouring out to me many of the things she has learned through counselling cancer patients. Without her, this book could not have been written.

INTRODUCTION

It was a beautiful wedding. The candles flickered, casting a warm glow through the pews filled with friends and loved ones. At the sound of the wedding march, all eyes turned to Jan. Her dark eyes were shining and happy, and Greg's heart beat faster as she neared. He saw the ivory satin gown she had spent hours making, lovingly stitching the lace around the bodice. She carried roses and daisies.

Neither of them knew then that Jan's life would be like the spring flowers in her hands—lovely, full of life, but gone far too soon.

Greg is my husband's brother. All of us in the family loved Jan from the time he first brought her home for us to meet. We were happy for them as we saw their love deepen and grow stronger. They planned for their marriage ceremony with joy and anticipation. They dreamed of a house and children and a lifetime together.

Not quite two years after the wedding, Jan became ill. Nausea, double vision, numbness in one arm. Was it flu? The headaches were unbearable. Was it nerves? Doctors were consulted, but they had trouble diagnosing the problem. Soon it became clear that something was seriously wrong. At last, surgery. Then an answer.

Diagnosis: brain tumour, malignant.

This lovely girl was not yet twenty-five. All her hopes for her future as a woman came crashing down around her. Her dreams of being the mother of a houseful of children were gone. As health ebbed from her, so did her physical beauty.

Every single *earthly* hope she ever had was snatched away from her.

As the rest of us stumbled through those long, agonising months, we saw the stark reality of human tragedy. We witnessed the anguish of her mother and father, the heartbreak Greg was suffering. We grieved with Jan as the days passed and the hope for recovery slipped away.

The feeling that seemed hardest to deal with was that of helplessness. As long as there was a surgery that might help or therapy that might help or drugs that might help, the feeling of impotence was lessened. But as these medical techniques, one by one, became less dependable, we all felt we were drowning in a sea of despair. This sense of helplessness, I learned, is part of the terror of terminal cancer.

We asked the questions.

Why God, why?

How could you do this awful thing to such a sweet girl whose life was just beginning?

I wanted so much to be able to ease the sense of hopelessness, but I felt inadequate. I ached with the desire to tell her of the confidence we might have in the God of the universe who is both sovereign—the blessed Controller of all things—and the one who loves us with an everlasting love. But I was just beginning to understand these things myself, so again I felt inadequate.

During the course of Jan's illness, I met an extraordinary woman named Nell Collins, who is both a nurse and a cancer patient. Nell was a head nurse at Community Hospital in Indianapolis. At the time I met her she was leaving that work to become a full-time missionary to cancer patients. Her work would take place primarily in Indiana, but she would often see patients in other states.

I heard Nell speak about her counselling ministry—about how God had directed her life in such a way that she was able to bring help and comfort to cancer patients.

Nell and I went to Dayton, Ohio, to see Jan. Though our visit was short, Jan was able to relate to Nell some of her doubts, fears, and frustrations. Nell spoke with Jan about our sovereign God, who cradles us in his everlasting arms.

I became interested in Nell's ministry. As time went on, I became more and more aware of the effect of cancer on people's lives. As a journalist, I began to see cancer as a phenomenon that seemed to touch everyone, either personally or in the life of a loved one, and I wrote several articles about Nell, her ministry, and the special needs of cancer patients.

Cancer is often called the most feared disease, and I do believe that description is true. We are all afraid of cancer. Jan was the victim of one of the most dreaded and devastating forms of cancer. Her neurosurgeon told us that the type of malignancy she had was extremely fast-growing and not one that ordinarily responds well to treatment. She lived about a year and a half after diagnosis.

Today, as never before, there is hope of cure for many forms of cancer. What Jan experienced is an example of what we all fear, but millions of people who have encountered the disease live many normal, active years after proper treatment, and a large number of those people are eventually pronounced cured.

Nevertheless, cancer wreaks havoc in the lives of its victims, family members, and friends. How can a person live with it? That is not an easy question, and I shall not for a minute suggest that I have all the answers. But God has given us some answers, and those answers can be discovered in the Bible.

My grandmother died with breast cancer before I was born. Daddy has often told me how she loved the Lord and her Bible and how much comfort she got from reading its well-worn pages. I believe the Bible's comfort was a reality for Nellie Mattox, and I believe comfort is there for us today.

Nell Collins has given me insight into the needs, hopes, and fears that a person with cancer may have. I am not a doctor or a theologian or a cancer patient. But God has been showing me the tremendous worry, fear, and heartbreak that often accompanies this particular disease.

Every time I read the statistics about the millions of people with cancer in this country, I know that each number represents a home gripped by the icy fingers of fear. Cancer, in its various forms, strikes one person in every three in this country at some time in their lives, and kills 150,000 people in Britain each year—many of them never knowing the true meaning of hope.

I began to see a need for a book for cancer patients, their families, loved ones, and others concerned about the lives touched by this particular disease. The aim of *Living with Cancer* is to explain in understandable terms some of the medical aspects of cancer, to face squarely examples of practical problems often encountered, to look honestly at the emotional responses experienced by the people involved, and to show clearly the tremendous hope and encouragement available to the Christian who faces this situation.

Cancer is not one disease; it is many. The type, location, and extent of the disease determines the seriousness of it. It is hoped that this book will help cancer patients in any situation. However, those people who are dealing with cancer of a less severe nature should not be discouraged or frightened by references to more serious problems. Each case is unique, and it would be unwise to compare one situation with another.

I have interviewed numerous cancer patients and their families. These people have had to deal with cancer of different types, and there has been a variety of outcomes. Each of them will speak through these pages.

Care will be taken to protect the identities of all the patients involved, and no real names will be used except those in this introduction and a few taken from published material. Some illustrations are fictional, but are typical of experiences encountered by real people. The use of any name that belongs to an actual person is a coincidence.

It is my prayer that "the peace of God, which passeth all understanding, shall keep your hearts and minds through Christ Jesus" (Phil. 4:7).

1

A VERY SPECIAL NURSE

"Cancer," says Nell Collins, "touches everybody. Either you've got it, or you're scared of getting it."

Nell knows about cancer.

Until more than a decade ago she knew about the disease from a strictly professional standpoint. She worked for nine years as head nurse in a constant care unit of a large American hospital. She was very familiar with cancer and what it can do to a person's body, mind, and spirit. At that time she helped people deal with the physical aspect of cancer as well as other illnesses requiring around-the-clock attention.

Nell led an exciting and enviable life. At twenty-nine, she was involved in a career she loved; she had high goals and great ambitions.

Then one day a mole on her back started changing.

That mole changed her life. It was cancer. Malignant melanoma.

"People who have not yet experienced it," says Nell, "do not know the horror of the moment when you are first told you have a malignancy growing in your body. I felt as if a death sentence had been stamped on my name."

During the initial hysteria, Nell screamed and cried; she was enveloped by disbelief and fear.

Then, for the first time in her young life, facing death, she began to consider life according to God's economy.

"I suddenly realised that the diagnosis of cancer was not necessarily my appointment with death. But it was that diagnosis that made me aware that every single human being does have that death appointment."

LIKE A TRAFFIC LIGHT

Nell compares life to observing traffic lights.

"Most of us", she says, "just go along our way. As long as we have the green light, we never even consider death, the red light. But when cancer has been diagnosed, the green light changes to yellow. With a jolt we are made aware that someday, whether from the cancer or a car accident or something else, the red light is going to come."

Since that fateful day several years ago, Nell has found the real meaning for her life, and in spite of the fact that she has had two operations for malignant melanoma and dozens of moles removed for biopsy, she has a joy and peace that she never before thought possible.

Early in life, Nell wanted to be a missionary in Africa. She went to a Bible college to prepare for that work. She could not understand why the doors kept closing and why she was not able to work as a missionary nurse. Now, of course, she knows.

"God had other plans for me," says Nell with a wry grin. "I had been a Christian for several years," she says, "and I knew the Bible had some very specific information concerning life and death. I had to lie on my stomach for weeks so the skin graft on my back could heal. As the days passed I studied God's Word with an intensity I'd never known before.

"As I recognised more and more just who God is, who man is, what sin is, and what righteousness really is—as I realised just how Christ paid for my sin, and how I can know God personally through faith in Christ—only then, without fear, did I turn my life over to Christ and give him complete control.

"Then there was peace in the midst of turmoil, joy in the face of sorrow, hopelessness turned to hope, and fear turned to trust."

In time Nell gave up her regular hospital nursing career to become a missionary to cancer patients. She has visited several thousand people who have encountered this disease. She knows of no other missionary/nurse working specifically with cancer patients and their families.

NELL RELATES TO PATIENTS

Emotionally, Nell can relate to cancer patients because she herself has had surgery and drug therapy for the disease.

"Often", she says, "it's the fact that I have had cancer surgery that enables a person to really open up with me."

Nell has found that cancer patients need a friend, somebody who really understands what they are going through.

"We're in the same boat", she says simply, "so they find it easy to relate to me. They row on their side, and I row on mine. But we're going through it together, and they know it. I can help them through the rough times because I've been there."

Nell feels that physical needs, for the most part, are recognised and treated. Science has, of necessity, concentrated on the physical side of the disease, trying to find a cure and ways to ease the pain. Emotional responses to those physical needs, though not so well understood, are getting more attention now than in previous years. Spiritual needs, however, are being virtually ignored.

"The modern world", says Nell, "has tried to deny man's spirituality, tried to pretend it doesn't exist. These people are in a face-to-face confrontation with the basic questions about the meaning of life. Most people know very little of what is in the Bible. They've been raised in a society that worships science and technology as the answer to all of life's problems. Their spirituality has been denied."

Nell has discovered that underlying many of the outward problems of the cancer patient is spiritual need: the need to know that God *is*; the need to know he cares in a personal way; the need to know he has provided a way to know him; the need to know he knows what is best and he is in control of everything—even when the situation seems an unmistakable tragedy from our point of view.

FEAR OF THE UNKNOWN

The fear of cancer is related, Nell believes, to a person's spiritual condition. This fear must be recognised.

Fear is a normal human reaction to the diagnosis of cancer. The fear, sometimes, is of the unknown. Cancer patients might be tortured by the following factors:

They do not know
1. what caused the cancer;
2. if surgery has been necessary, has the surgeon got it all;
3. if they will have to suffer a lot of pain, and if so, if they will be able to handle it;
4. how it will affect their physical appearance;
5. if it has spread (metastasised) to another location in the body;
6. what effect it will have on their children, or if the children will become overly worried about their own bodies;
7. if they will be a burden to their families;
8. which treatment will work best;
9. how their bodies will react to treatment, or what side effects they might have;

10. how long they will live;
11. if the people around them are telling them the truth, or if they are trying to hide something from them (they are suspicious of everyone);
12. how much money this whole thing will cost;
13. if they will be able to continue to work, or if they will become dependent;
14. if their partners will still love them and stand beside them;
15. what dying is like, or if there is life after death.

And the fear settles deep within. A young man with advanced lung cancer could hardly breathe, but he expressed the fear common to cancer patients: "I'm scared. I'm scared of dying. I'm scared of living. I'm scared of the cancer."

Regardless of the type of cancer or its location in the body, Nell says that a cancer patient never again can look at life or death from the same perspective he had before.

Because of the cancer, his life will be different from the way it was before the diagnosis. He wishes with all his heart that he could go back to those days when cancer was something that happened to somebody else. But he cannot.

Cancer, no matter what the prognosis, is a fact in his life. He must live with it.

2

CELLS GONE BERSERK

Terror clutched her heart the moment Alice Johnson heard the voice on the telephone.

"This is Dr Adams," he said, "and I'm just really sorry to have to call you like this."

He did not have to tell her. She knew by the sadness in his voice that he had the report from the biopsy. Bad news.

Feeling hot and cold all at once, she seemed to be watching the scene on TV in slow motion.

". . . malignant . . . schedule surgery right away . . ."

She heard only snatches of what he was saying.

"Do you want me to call Don and tell him?"

"No—no, that's all right," she heard herself saying. "I can tell him." *Don! The kids! How will they take it?*

Her hands were shaking hard; it was all she could do to write down the information the doctor was giving her.

Afterwards, she looked without seeing at the clutter in the kitchen; breakfast dishes were stacked all over. She heard herself screaming. *My life is over*, she thought.

Cancer.

THE FEARFUL DIAGNOSIS

Has anyone ever heard this diagnosis without fear, without panic? Like Nell and millions of others, Alice suddenly felt a cloud of doom over her life. She was in the "valley of the shadow of death", and for the first time in her life she understood the real meaning of fear.

"I was terrified," said Alice. "I began imagining aches and pains all over my body, and I was convinced that the cancer had spread everywhere. I just knew that I was going to die, and soon. Like within a few weeks.

"I was terrified of the pain that I might have to endure. My grandmother died with cancer, and I remembered how she suffered.

"And my pride—oh, how that hurt. I had always been so proud. Secretly, I think I felt I was a little better than other people.

"I mean, something like that just couldn't happen to me. After all, I had been a beauty queen in college! I was married to a wonderful guy, and I had always had everything I wanted—even what I thought was the perfect family—one boy, one girl.

"Then, suddenly, I was faced with cancer. It was a humbling experience, believe me. *Me*, with cancer! I just couldn't believe it could happen to me. I guess I thought I was above it."

NO RESPECTER OF PERSONS

As Alice found out, cancer is no respecter of persons. It strikes young, old, rich, poor, all races and religions, beauty queens and wallflowers. People in all parts of the world have it in some form.

Cancer is not even limited to people. Dogs and cats get it. Wild animals, reptiles, plants, and insects all can get cancer.

The Cancer Research Campaign reports that about one million British people are in treatment for cancer at any one time. Over the years, cancer will strike one person in every three.[1]

Nearly everyone, it seems, will encounter cancer some-day, either personally or in the life of a loved one. But today we can have a real hope for cure.

There are over five million Americans alive today who have a history of cancer, three million of them with a diagnosis five or more years ago. Most of these three million can be considered cured. One out of three people treated for cancer now has a normal life expectancy.

Great advances have been made in the treatments for cancers, especially certain types. Hodgkin's disease, Wilms' tumour, acute lymphocytic leukaemia, and testicular cancer are among those cancers that are treated with more promis-ing results than ever before.

FIRST IDENTIFIED 400 BC

Man has been fighting cancer since before Hippocrates first identified it about 400 BC. He divided tumours into two large groups, the "innocuous" (or benign) and "dangerous" (or malignant). He also coined the term *karkinoma* (meaning "crab") for solid, malignant tumours. The Latin word for "crab," *cancrum*, was later the basis for our word *cancer*. No one is sure why Hippocrates chose the word *crab* to describe malignant tumours, but some people guess it is because the crab grabs hold of its prey with such tenacity.

Until this century there was little hope for the cancer patient; death was inevitable. Today the outlook is much brighter. With early diagnosis and proper treatment, more and more people are saved from cancer every year. Using chemotherapy, surgery, and radiotherapy, either as a single treatment or in sophisticated combinations with other measures, cancer is now considered one of the most curable diseases in this country.

Surgery is one of the most significant treatments for the disease, and it is always recommended wherever possible.

Radiotherapy effectively stops the growth of cancer cells in certain types of cancers. About half of all cancer patients are treated with radiation, either alone or in combination with other therapy.

Beyond these two measures, cancer is now being successfully treated by radioactive substances, various drugs, chemicals, and hormones. The treatment of cancer is extremely complex, but basically the intent is to remove cancer cells by surgery or to destroy them (or inhibit reproduction) with radiation or chemotherapy.

The physician might hope to bring about a *remission*, which is a temporary state wherein the symptoms of the disease are not manifested. Being in remission is not the same as being cured, because the cancer cells are still in the body, even if they cannot be seen through a microscope.

Today, doctors and patients alike are frustrated because for centuries this disease has defied researchers to find an absolute cause or a positive cure. One reason for the difficulty in dealing with this disease is that there are more than 150 recognisable kinds of cancer, each with its own problems and patterns of behaviour.

When cancer is diagnosed, the patient might come under the care of a haematologist/oncologist. Haematology is the study of the blood; oncology is the study of tumours.

WHAT IS IT, ANYWAY?

The word *cancer* is used to describe an uncontrolled growth of abnormal cells. A body is made up of billions of normal cells, all of which multiply and divide in an orderly manner to perform their own particular functions. Whenever these cells, for some as yet unknown reason, go berserk and grow in a disorderly and chaotic manner, crowding out normal cells and robbing them of nourishment, the condition is known as cancer. The disease creeps into a life insidiously, normally without pain until it is advanced.

Some cancers are more serious than others. Some are fast-growing; some are slow-growing. In fact there is no set rate of growth. Some types grow more in a few weeks than others grow in several years. Cancer can start in any tissue of the body.

Some are discovered early, before they have spread. Others are located in places in the body where surgery and radiotherapy are difficult, if not impossible. In many sites, however, cancer is curable by these techniques if detected early.

Cancer is a group of diseases in which there is uncontrolled growth of abnormal cells, which, if unchecked, will cause death. Because of this fact, it is important that surgery and other recommended treatments are not delayed.

Though researchers have been trying to find the causes of the disease, the task is difficult because cancer behaves in so many different ways. Some cancers have been induced in animals by viruses; this has led scientists to believe that in the future it might be possible to vaccinate against a few forms of the disease. More and more convincing evidence is becoming available that in many cases cancer is environmentally induced.

USUALLY DEFINED BY SITE

Each type of cancer is normally defined by the place, or site, in the body where it is growing. The appendix in this book contains detailed information on the most frequent sites of the disease in humans. Cancer is further defined by the biological characteristics of the tumour. It should be noted, again, that not all tumours are malignant. A benign tumour, though abnormal, is rarely dangerous to a person's life. It grows to a certain size and then stops growing; it does not spread.

A malignant (cancerous) tumour, on the other hand, keeps on growing. The cells from the original site of the cancer can dislodge, be carried by the bloodstream or lymphatic systems to other parts of the body, and give rise to additional tumours. This spreading of cancer is called *metastasis*. Without treatment, these tumours will eventually invade vital organs, robbing them of nourishment and causing death.

A physician suspicious of cancer will order a number of tests, but the most accurate test used is the biopsy. In this test a sample of tissue is removed and examined chemically and microscopically.

MOST PEOPLE CLING TO HOPE

Until the diagnosis is confirmed, most people cling to the hope that it will not be cancer.

"Of all people, being a nurse," says Nell Collins, "I should have been suspicious that that mole might have been a malignant melanoma. But I refused to let the idea enter my mind. I wouldn't let myself believe the possibility existed that I might have cancer. I went to have the biopsy done, never really considering that it might be cancer."

Another woman, Wilma Kirk, was preparing to enter the hospital to have a lump removed from her breast. She was hoping it would not be cancer, but found herself relying on totally worthless facts.

"Sometimes," Wilma says, "just to have hope, we grasp at straws. When I went into the hospital, I was in a five-bed room, all of us there for breast biopsies. Out of all the other women, only one of the biopsies was malignant, and that was an elderly lady.

"I grabbed on to that fact for hope. I told myself that this could only happen to old people. Then one of the nurses told me that I had a lucky bed, that everyone who had that bed got to go home the next day. So that, again, gave me hope. Funny how we put our confidence in things like that."

Wilma woke up after surgery with the breast and muscle tissue removed, her hopes in the "lucky bed" and in her quite erroneous calculation that "it only happens to old people" completely destroyed.

When she realised what had happened, she screamed hysterically, ripping the bandages off and pulling out the drainage tubes. At that moment her grief was beyond words.

Ten years have passed in Wilma's life since that terrible day. She will never forget the panic she felt in those first moments, but because of her relationship with Christ, she has adjusted to the fact of cancer in her life. Through Reach to Recovery, a rehabilitation programme of the American Cancer Society designed to meet the special needs of mastectomy patients, she is now helping others facing the loss of a breast. (If you have had breast surgery or are now facing it, write to the Mastectomy Association of Great Britain, 26 Harrison Street, Off Gray's Inn Road, King's Cross, WC1H 8JG. Tel: 01-837 0908. Or contact Reach for Recovery which operates in Scotland and Ireland, c/o The Secretary, 'Crosswinds', 2 Earl Grey Street, Tollcross, Edinburgh, Scotland.)

Once the diagnosis of cancer has been made, a person should not be surprised if the response to that diagnosis is great fear and anxiety. Nearly everyone reacts to the very word *cancer* with dread. Sometimes a person may try to fight the fear with bravado, but underneath remains a disquieting apprehension concerning the unknown future.

3

SELF-ESTEEM AND
THE CANCER PATIENT

What is it that gives a person a sense of worth? Of value as a human being?

Psychologists have spent long years studying the phenomenon of self-esteem in an effort to determine the factors involved in a person's opinion of himself.

The factors are many and varied. They involve such attributes as physical appearance, intelligence, character, the ability to work and be productive, and the ability to compensate for real or imagined shortcomings.

The cancer patient's opinion of himself, either consciously or unconsciously, will be threatened in some way by the disease. His physical appearance may be altered by surgery or other treatment, causing a change in the way he looks and the way he views himself—his "body image". His intelligence will probably not be affected, unless there is a direct attack on the central nervous system. However, he may find that suddenly people are treating him as though he were a child, and not a very bright one at that. If he wants to discuss real fears, he may get a patronising response. Deep-seated fears and smouldering anger, causing him to question his strength of character, might be brought out by the diagnosis.

Of course, a tremendous amount of self-esteem revolves around the ability to work and be productive. Getting back to work or normal daily routine is very important to most cancer patients. If a person is physically limited so that he cannot return to his former activities, it is extremely important that he find something to do instead to compensate for his loss.

ONE WOMAN'S BATTLE

Elizabeth Ann Tierney, a treatment-room nurse on Head and Neck Service, reports in *American Journal of Nursing* the case of one woman's battle against cancer. She tells about Eileen, a woman in her middle fifties who came to be treated for extensive oral cancer.

"Eileen", she says, "had an infiltrating epidermoid cancer on the left gingiva. Because epithelial tissue is so abundant in the oral cavity, this kind of cancer can be widely disseminated there. The evaluation at Memorial revealed no metastatic sites." (What this meant was that Eileen had wide-spread cancer in her gums and in the tissue lining the mouth, but it had not spread to another part of her body.)

After conferences with Eileen, the doctors decided that control could be achieved with a mandibulectomy (removal of the lower jaw), total glossectomy (complete removal of the tongue), resection of the floor of the mouth, and bilateral neck node dissection. The radical procedure would impair her swallowing, breathing, and speech; convalescence would require lengthy and painful adjustments.[1]

Eileen had to face fears connected with the purely physical aspects of the surgery, the most pronounced anxieties surrounding her inability to communicate and the fear of asphyxiation.

But beyond these things, Eileen's sense of self-esteem would be under brutal attack. She realised, of course, that the cancer, if left alone, would in time cause damage equally as extensive as that of the surgery. The alternatives to the surgery—haemorrhage, suffocation, pain, and death—helped put the need for the surgery into perspective. So she decided to go ahead. The surgery was done successfully, and after a difficult adjustment period she began looking forward to the time when she could undergo reconstructive plastic surgery.

PHYSICAL BEAUTY

Eileen's opinion of herself had to have been affected tremendously by this experience. Why? Because not only was her body image changed, but the alteration was in a place that could not be concealed.

James Dobson, Ph.D, says, "Without question, the most highly valued personal attribute in our culture (and in most others) is physical attractiveness."[2]

We cannot escape the emphasis our culture places on beauty—sheer, physical, skin-deep beauty. If we cannot be beautiful, our culture then insists that we at least not be "disfigured" or "abnormal" or "different" in any way.

This cultural emphasis on physical perfection is one of the first concerns of the cancer patient. He asks, "What will happen to my body?" He may not ask the question verbally, but it is there.

Breast cancer has been the object of a great amount of publicity in America mainly because of the national attention given the wives of several political figures who talked openly about their mastectomies. Their frankness has been instrumental in partially removing the cloak of secrecy that has in the past surrounded breast cancer.

Rene C. Mastrovito, MD, explains how mastectomy surgery is more devastating for some women than others:

The psychological assault of a radical mastectomy is greater on some women than it is on others. A woman whose concept of self-worth is significantly and strongly dependent upon her sense of femininity and her female body image will have suffered a greater loss than will a woman whose personal identification makes this attribute less important.[3]

Though we all have great concern for our bodies, we must remember that in God's economy real beauty is seen in a heart that is in right relationship with him. He loves us and accepts us as we are, inside and out.

EMOTIONAL RESPONSE

Any drastic change in body image caused by the cancer or the accompanying treatment will cause an emotional response on the part of the patient. Just the fact of cancer, by itself, causes an emotional reaction. This emotional response may or may not be expressed verbally.

Eileen Tiedt in *Nursing Forum* says, "Our society places an enormous stigma on cancer . . . Because of the stigma attached to cancer and the value placed on the intact, healthy body, cancer patients do not readily talk about what has and is happening to them." She says that the patient's emotional energy is spent helping others to cope with their emotional response to the patient's situation. The patient thus uses energy needed to cope with his own needs.[4]

One exceptionally healthy-looking man in the prime of life chooses to tell no one other than his wife about his cancer. He knows of the stigma attached to the disease, and he wants no one to treat him differently or with pity. As Rene Mastrovito says:

> Cancer is a source of severe psychological as well as somatic [bodily] stress. It is a feared disease because it implies a fatal outcome. It is a dreaded disease because of projected fears of pain, body damage, deterioration and invalidism. It is a repugnant disease because it imbues the victim with a certain sense of being unclean and unwholesome. Finally it is a condition that may

engender an overpowering sense of helplessness because, contrary to their attitudes about many other serious illnesses, cancer patients feel that there is little or nothing that they can do in their own defence. In many, cancer is a catastrophic phenomenon; it is unforeseen, ravaging and, if it does not destroy completely, it leaves in its wake losses which cannot easily be replaced.[5]

A person's self-esteem is vitally affected by his emotional responses to difficult or life-threatening circumstances.

Maurice E. Wagner, Th.M, Ph.D, describes the stress that a person might encounter when he is given a diagnosis of cancer:

> Our self-concept may seem fairly stable when life's ebb and flow of problems stays within acceptable limits. Occasionally, however, a tidal wave of unexpected difficulties overwhelms us. It may be a surprise illness, the sudden death of a loved one, a business failure, or a marriage or family problem we cannot handle. Our boat is not only rocked: it seems as if it is about to split in the middle and take water.[6]

COPING MECHANISMS

Just to get along in day-to-day life we all use what psychiatrists refer to as "coping mechanisms". These are, Mastrovito says, various "strategies, behaviour patterns, attitudes, and personal physical and emotional attributes which are used in dealing with one's self and environment. Where successful, these life patterns maintain self-esteem, acceptability by others and a sense of mastery over one's destiny."[7]

You will notice that physical attributes are mentioned among the coping mechanisms that are important to a sense of worthiness or self-esteem. If a physical attribute is changed or removed due to the cancer, the patient has lost an important psychological coping mechanism.

Of course, each person's situation is unique, and it is
difficult to make generalisations about cancer. A simple,
isolated, and uncomplicated cancer might be removed
completely and cause the patient no further distress. Others
might experience the tremendous stress of catastrophe.
Tiedt sees the varying emotional needs thus:

> From a psychological point of view, the emotional needs and
> responses of all involved with the patient with cancer will
> depend on the specific nature of the cancer, its site, its treatment,
> and its course; these will determine to what the patient and
> family must adjust. Some cancers have the likelihood of
> violating the patient's self-image, such as skin lesions or scars
> resulting in amputation, and bowel or renal lesions resulting
> in a type of stomy. Other cancers imply an imminent life-
> threatening catastrophe, such as gross, central nervous system
> changes which may cause paralysis, blindness, or vital disturb-
> ance.[8]

What coping mechanisms are used by the cancer patient?

Denial. Probably every cancer patient, at one time or
another, uses the coping mechanism of *denial*. Denial is an
unconscious process used to some degree by all of us in
everyday life. Not everyone, of course, uses denial in the
same way.

"Denial", says Mastrovito, "is not necessarily a patholo-
gical condition. Since it is a protective mechanism, it can
frequently serve the individual well in preventing overwhelming anxiety or marked depression."[9]

Often, however, denial is not healthy. In fact, it may
ignore or distort reality.

The first place where denial might come into play for the
cancer patient is before diagnosis. He has a symptom that
he knows to be one of the warning signs of cancer, but he
denies that possibility and does not seek medical care.

When diagnosis is finally made, denial is put to work
again. "There must have been some mistake," says the

patient. "Maybe the laboratory got the names mixed up." The patient may go from doctor to doctor in an effort to disprove the diagnosis.

As the disease progresses, all of the negative information is minimised, and the positive information is emphasised. Physicians commonly encourage this sort of denial, thinking they must maintain hope as long as possible. There is a fine line between having a positive attitude and denying reality.

A cancer patient who is trusting Christ for every detail of his life does not need to deny reality. "Behold, Thou dost desire truth in the innermost being, and in the hidden part Thou wilt make me know wisdom" (Ps. 51:6).

In this psalm, David is praying for forgiveness, but I believe the verse also can be applied to denial. God wants us to face reality and to know the truth. He does not want us to pretend that cancer does not exist when it does. Being realistic means that the person sees the situation as it really is—no worse and no better.

Accepting help. It is often a severe trial for the cancer patient's self-esteem to simply accept help.

Betty Olsen, the mother of three active preschoolers at the time of diagnosis, was accustomed to her busy routine: caring for the children, cleaning, cooking. She thoroughly enjoyed her home and family and loved gardening and making preserves. She took pride in doing things herself.

The diagnosis of uterine cancer did not have much effect on Betty's self-esteem at first.

"I was just so relieved to have the tumour removed", she said, "that I didn't think too much about it. I can remember thinking I was glad, at least, that it was in the uterus instead of the breast. At least the surgery didn't show!

"But I had to go back into the hospital later for a rather vigorous round of therapy, and I had to be away from my husband and kids for three weeks. While I was at the hospital, I kept imagining how terrible it was for them. I had always done everything for everybody—they even needed me to pick out their clothes every day.

"When I got home, I was shocked. I was weak and didn't feel very well, but I had enough strength to simmer with anger.

"Why, it didn't look like they had missed me one bit! I'd never seen the house so clean, and the kids were all making their own beds and picking out their own clothes to wear! I knew I should have been happy about them getting along so well, but I guess my pride was hurt. Instead of being happy, I was really resentful."

As Betty's bout with cancer stretched over several years, accepting help became more and more of a problem for her.

"My neighbours," she says, "were very good at bringing in food and taking the children every time I had a problem. And I really do appreciate everything they've done—we couldn't have made it without them.

"But, after a while, I began to get really depressed because I realised that everyone was doing everything for me, and there was no way I could possibly repay them."

Being able to accept help from others is often very difficult for the cancer patient. Knowing he *needs* help adds to the feelings of helplessness and vulnerability.

The problem of accepting help is tied strongly to the patient's intense desire to be "normal" and not to be different from anyone else. Because there might be times when he is totally dependent on others to help him, his self-esteem can be badly bruised.

Remembering the patient's fragile self-esteem, family and friends should offer help in a gentle, sensitive way. The patient should be encouraged to do as much as he possibly can. Self-esteem can be boosted, too, by asking the patient his advice or asking for his opinion regarding a problem you might have. People who have suffered difficulties often have great depth of character and can often give excellent counsel.

Compensation. The concept of compensation is important for everybody's self-esteem, but has particular meaning to the cancer patient. A person compensates by counterbalancing his shortcomings with a concentration on his strengths.

This concept is beautifully illustrated by the story of Joni Eareckson Tada who, as an athletic teenager, had a diving accident and became a quadriplegic. Her self-esteem had centred largely on her athletic ability: horseback riding, waterskiing, swimming. Her diving accident took away the ability to use her arms and legs. She went through periods of great despair before she began to lean totally on Christ. Eventually, she discovered that her talent for drawing, which she had enjoyed before the accident, was not confined to her useless hands. By learning to draw with a pen in her mouth, she developed this talent amazingly. By *compensating* in this way, she found both a means of expression and a rewarding career.

It is important for any person who has endured physical limitations because of cancer to look for an area that he can develop to compensate for his loss.

Bear one another's burdens. Another means of maintaining or restoring self-esteem is found in the Christian commandment to "bear one another's burdens." Dobson describes the psychological effect:

> This same Christian principle offers the most promising solution to *your* inferiority and inadequacy, as well. I have repeatedly observed that a person's needs and problems seem less threatening when he is busy helping someone else handle theirs. It is difficult to wallow in your own troubles when you are actively shouldering another person's load and seeking solutions to his problems. For each discouraged reader who feels unloved and

shortchanged by life, I would recommend that you consciously make a practice of giving to others. Visit the sick. Bake something for your neighbour. Use your car for those without transportation. And perhaps most importantly, learn to be a good listener. The world is filled with lonely, disheartened people like yourself, and you are in an excellent position to empathise with them. And while you're doing it, I guarantee that your own sense of uselessness will begin to fade.[10]

This concept was put into practice by a woman who, because of massive surgery for cancer, was forced to quit her job of over thirty years. Thinking that she was totally useless, she was swallowed up in despair.

"I was not married", she says, "and I had no family. My life revolved around my career. Suddenly my daily routine no longer existed; my financial status changed greatly. This left a feeling of uselessness. I got so depressed I didn't care if I lived or not.

"One night when I was extremely depressed, I rang Nell Collins. She knew something was wrong. She asked me if I had Christ in my heart, and I said no. So it was right there on the phone that I prayed to receive Christ. My problems did not disappear, and I still had times of great depression. But Nell kept counselling me and showing me what God says in his Word. I finally realised that everything that had happened was in God's will for me."

This woman slowly began to see God's love and plan for her life. As time went on, she started helping Nell by typing letters and taking care of some other paperwork. As Nell's mission field expanded, so did her secretarial needs, and a woman who had thought of herself as useless became the "right arm" of Nell's ministry.

"For the first time in my life", she says, "I have *real* purpose and meaning to my life. Through all those years in government service, my life really had no meaning at all. But now I know that my life does have a purpose that's real and eternal, and I thank God for the cancer."

We cannot truly understand our real value in terms of earthly things: beauty, intelligence, talent. To see our real worth we must begin to understand the price that God paid to bring us to himself. Our redemption was costly—the precious blood of Jesus, his own Son. There is no greater love than this. That God himself came to this planet in human form to suffer and die for us gives us an idea of what God must consider our true worth to be.

4

SPECIAL PROBLEMS

Cancer does not always mean a change in life-style. A cancer patient often is able to return to work and other daily activities without the treatment for cancer greatly affecting his day-to-day routine.

Radical surgery, of course, can cause serious problems of adjustment. Patients with colon-rectum cancer may need to adjust to wearing a colostomy bag; breast cancer surgery usually involves the loss of the breast and surrounding tissue. Laryngectomees often need to learn to talk without vocal cords, and sometimes bone cancer patients must lose an arm or leg and then learn to use an artificial limb.

These problems are real, and most people who have surgery that changes the body image or function will go through a period of great distress and depression. If the cancer patient has lost a part of his body, he will mourn that loss. His grief will be much like that which he would experience if a loved one had died. The loss is permanent.

As Christians, we know that these physical bodies are only temporary dwelling places. We know that someday God will give us each a new, resurrected body, which will be perfect in every respect. That does comfort us. But while living here in a physical body, one naturally will be distressed if a part of that body is lost. It is hard to imagine getting along without it.

One salesman said, "I knew I had to lose my vocal cords in order to live—I just wasn't sure I wanted to live without my vocal cords. After all, my business, my livelihood, depended on my ability to talk." After long and difficult months of training, he has now learned oesophageal speech and is adjusting to his loss.

Many people do have limitations of this kind thrust on them within a few days or hours of diagnosis. The result of the cancer is visible and drastic. It is even more of a shock because the symptoms had often seemed barely significant enough to call to the doctor's attention. One woman said, "I just couldn't believe that tiny lump could change things so drastically."

Surgery for cancer sometimes must be extensive and radical to remove all tissue to which the cancer may have spread. In *Science against Cancer*, Pat McGrady says that surgical techniques, enhanced by new anaesthetics, more effective antibiotics to control infection, transfusions, and rigid sterile precautions are now permitting operative procedures that would have been impossible a few years ago.[1]

RADIOTHERAPY

In radiation, too, remarkable strides have been made. Such instruments as linear accelerators, betatrons, and radioactive cobalt-60 teletherapy apparatus have become standard equipment for treating deep-seated cancers.

Radiotherapy uses ionising radiations to destroy cells by injuring their capacity to divide. Some cancers are more responsive to radiation than others. The new radiation instruments produce energy in the multi-million electron volt range and can deliver a greater dose of radiation to deep-seated tumours without the discomfort and skin reactions that often accompany the lower-energy X-ray beams.

PROBLEMS WITH CHEMOTHERAPY

Twenty-five years ago, chemotherapy was reserved for the cancer patient with widespread metastases and little hope of recovery. It was a last-ditch effort.

Today, chemotherapy plays a major role in the early treatment of cancer. It is a standard form of therapy, and oncologists use it routinely with the goal of curing the patient.

Susan Golden in *Nursing Forum* gives the reason for the optimism: "Three major advances in cancer chemotherapy have contributed to this new perspective: (1) the development of new drugs, (2) the concept of combined-agent chemotherapy, and (3) the use of drug therapy in conjunction with radiation and surgery for early cancer patients with poor prognosis."

She notes that doctors have a choice of at least eighty anti-tumour drugs available, while new drugs are being developed steadily.[2]

The drugs used in chemotherapy act in two basic ways: they either kill tumour cells (cytocidal), or else they create conditions adverse to cell reproduction (cytostatic). These drugs are used with an exact knowledge of the cell cycle to get the maximum destruction of malignant cells at the varying stages of cell growth, while at the same time doing as little damage as possible to normal cells. Inevitably, though, normal cells will also be affected by the chemotherapy, and various side effects will result.

The drugs used in chemotherapy are designed to destroy the rapidly reproducing cancer cells. Therefore, the normal cells that naturally reproduce quickly will usually be the ones adversely affected by the drugs. The digestive tract, hair roots, and bone marrow all have actively reproducing cells; this is why it is common for patients on chemotherapy to lose their hair and have nausea, diarrhoea, mouth and lip ulcers, and blood-related problems (anaemia, insufficient white cell count, haemorrhage, etc.).

Not everyone has side effects, and sometimes these discomforts last just a few days. If the reaction to the drug is very severe, the physician may want to reduce the dosage or discontinue the drug altogether.

Hair loss. Hair loss can occur from both radiation and certain drugs used in chemotherapy. This is one of the most devastating side effects of treatment, and it is especially difficult for teenagers and young adults. This side effect is not dangerous, but it can be emotionally upsetting. It is important to understand that the drug or radiation is necessary in order to stop the growth of the cancer cells. The patient should be prepared well in advance so that he or she will know what is probably going to happen.

It is good to talk about getting a wig early, and a trip should be made to the barber shop or beauty salon before the loss is complete. Wigs are so common now for both men and women that a selection can be made with relative ease from any large department store. Eyebrow pencils and false eyelashes can also be purchased. Wigs can be obtained through the NHS either free (as an in-patient) or at reduced prices. The hair does grow back again after therapy, but it takes several months.

Weakness. Many cancer patients experience unusual lack of energy after radiation or chemotherapy. To people who are normally vibrant, this weakness is especially frustrating.

One working mother says: "It's all I can do to get through the day at work—I'm just so worn out. Then I come home and look around and see all the dust, and the Hoovering needs to be done, and I just feel like giving up. My husband

and the girls are great about pitching in and helping, but it still frustrates me that I can't do it myself. I'd also like to have company over for dinner sometimes, but I never know if I'll feel up to it, so we just never invite anyone."

GOD'S PROMISE

The treatment of cancer often causes difficult problems. Sometimes the problems seem just too much to bear; but God has promised that he has not given us anything to bear that other people have not endured before us, that he will not give us more than we can tolerate, and that he will provide the grace we need to get through especially rough times.

Our Lord Jesus Christ understands our sufferings. While he was here on earth, he too felt agony.

"For we have not an high priest which cannot be touched with the feeling of our infirmities; but was in all points tempted like as we are, yet without sin. Let us therefore come boldly unto the throne of grace, that we may obtain mercy, and find grace to help in time of need" (Heb. 4:15, 16).

5

FAMILY IN TURMOIL

Cancer does not strike in a vacuum. Not only is the patient affected, but also every member of the family: children, parents, brothers, sisters, husband or wife. The relationships of the family members are all put under severe stress.

Carole's husband cannot handle the fact that she has cancer. He gets drunk every time she has a doctor's appointment. He will not allow her or anyone else to talk about her illness. The children see the tremendous strain, their mother's tears, their father's unresolved anger; but they do not understand. They have not been told about the cancer.

George, a twenty-four-year-old bachelor, was living a swinging life when his bone cancer was diagnosed. After his arm was amputated, he moved back home with his parents. Though now all under one roof, the family is ripped apart by feelings of guilt, resentment, fear, and despair.

Jack is the pastor of a large church in the American Midwest. His father, who lives several states away, was diagnosed as having colon-rectum cancer and is not expected to live long. Jack feels strain from being too far away to help and guilt from not being there when needed.

Gloria found Christ because of a nurse who witnessed to her while she was in the hospital having cancer surgery. A mature woman with grown children, she is a baby

Christian. When she went home, her husband made fun of her decision. Her children and husband continue in their old habit patterns of cynicism and unbelief. As her health is failing more and more, the family is giving her less and less comfort. Her husband is jealous of her faith, and he causes her much unhappiness.

Herman, a young man with a wife and two small children, was diagnosed as having terminal lung cancer. How can the children be told that their daddy is going to die?

FAMILY TRAUMA

The entire family unit, close friends, and relatives suffer a certain degree of trauma when a dear one is diagnosed as having cancer. Of course, the severity of the trauma is directly related to the prognosis of the disease. If the outlook is good, and the surgery has not made a radical change in body image or function, the family problems are naturally lessened. The more problems and complications accompanying the cancer, the more traumatic it is for everyone concerned.

Chapter six deals with the special problems of childhood cancer; here, however, we shall discuss the questions most frequently asked concerning the family problems of an adult with cancer.

A diagnosis of cancer brings many questions from all family members. The questions concerning the medical aspects of the disease should be asked of the physician in charge of the case. I suggest you write out a list before you see your doctor so you can be sure every question is answered. Some doctors are very helpful about explaining everything in detail; others offer very little without being questioned. But if they know you really want to have it all explained to you, they will give you the answers you want.

Remember, however, that some questions cannot be answered. If he does not know, the doctor will say so.

In dealing with the family situation, the following questions are the ones I have heard most frequently. I have talked with doctors, nurses, patients, and family members to find answers.

Should small children be told that a parent has cancer?
Children have an amazing capacity to deal with truth. They will be hurt far more in the long run if you try to keep the illness a secret from them. If they do not find out from you, they will hear from someone else. Whispers and huddled conferences cause children more alarm than does the truth.

Of course, the *way* you tell them is extremely important. It will do them no good for you to be overly emotional, hysterical, or in a state of despair. It might be best to ask the doctor to explain to the children what is happening in a medical sense if you are too upset to do so.

If the children are quite young, you might tell them something like this: "Mummy found that she had something growing in her body that wasn't supposed to be there. It is called a tumour. The doctors had to remove the tumour, because it was very dangerous for it to be there. The tumour is sometimes called *cancer.* This is a very scary word, because sometimes people die when they have this kind of tumour growing in their bodies. Doctors now know a great deal more than they used to about taking care of people who have this happen." If the prognosis is good, say, "We think Mummy is going to be just fine."

Children should be given some specific information about the particular medical treatment, but should not be overburdened with too many details. They should be told the truth in a matter-of-fact manner. Above all, do not lie to the children. Do not tell them that Mummy has flu or some other minor problem. Tell them that the doctors are doing everything they can. Do not be afraid to say, I don't know.

If the disease gets progressively worse, tell the children that Mummy might not be able to get well. Reassure them that they will be loved, cared for, and not abandoned. Listen carefully to the questions they ask, and answer as simply and honestly as you can.

Telling the children about the serious illness of a parent, though very difficult, can be an opportunity to express to them your faith in a God who makes no mistakes. Memory of the way you trust Christ now will remain with your children the rest of their lives. Do not miss this opportunity to show them faith at work. Remember, do not exclude the children, thinking that you are protecting them. This time together can be precious.

What if the parent dies? If the parent should die, it is important that the child be allowed to grieve. This may seem obvious, but often in the midst of their own grief, family members will say things like, "You must be a big, brave boy now." This makes the child feel he cannot show emotion, so he keeps it all bottled up inside. Let him know it is all right for him to feel sad and to miss his parent.

Children often feel a tremendous sense of guilt because of the death of a parent. If the parent was ill at home, the child was probably told to keep quiet so the parent could rest. If the parent then dies, the child might conclude that he was not quiet enough, that he was responsible for the death. Help the child to discuss openly these fears and guilt feelings.

One little girl might be saddled for life with guilt feelings about her mother's death. Dorothy, aged thirty-two, just was not feeling well, but nothing very specific seemed to be wrong. At last she went to the hospital for tests. Diagnosis: cancer of the liver. She died within three weeks.

Her little girl was six years old. An aunt came to stay with her while her mother was in the hospital. The aunt repeatedly said to others in front of the little girl, "Dorothy never had any problems until *that girl* was born." It is highly unlikely that the cancer had any connection whatsoever with the birth of the little girl six years before, and no one knows what caused the aunt to reach this conclusion. The point, however, is that the child heard these remarks and very likely believed herself responsible for her mother's death. Be very careful what you say when tender little ones are around—even when you think they are not listening.

Should children go to the funeral of a parent? I believe that children over three years of age should be permitted to attend the funeral and burial of a loved one. It is hard if the child's first encounter with death is that of a parent, but he needs to be included in these ceremonies. The experience of the funeral is important in helping the living, including children, come to terms with the fact of death.

"I feel very blessed," said one young mother to me just a few weeks before she died. "I'm so glad I can talk about my death with my children. I can tell them that when they see my body at the funeral home, they'll be seeing just the shell. The 'real me' will not be there. The real me will be with Jesus. And, someday, when God says the time is right, we'll be reunited in that wonderful place! Isn't that great? If I had died suddenly in a car accident or something, we'd never have had the blessing of these precious times together."

What about parents of grown children who have cancer? What should their role be? Parents of an adult with cancer can be a real blessing or can cause tremendous stress. If there are young children needing care, grandparents can be a great help.

Be available; be sensitive. Offer help in a way so that your grown child can maintain self-esteem. Do not make him or her feel incapable.

Be extra sensitive to the needs of your child's husband or wife. You may have to step aside and let the spouse make decisions you feel entitled to make. You may not agree with every decision the spouse makes, but it is, nevertheless, his or her decision.

Mothers can sometimes tremendously upset grown daughters who have cancer by hovering and being emotionally distraught. The daughter then feels guilty about causing her mother so much grief. Also, the daughter can see right through it if the mother is putting up a front. The mother's visits should not be extremely long while her daughter is in the hospital recovering from surgery, because they might be emotionally tiring for her.

I feel I should be at the hospital every minute. If I have something come up that keeps me from visiting, I feel terribly guilty. What about this? It is important for close family members to keep a balance during a time of hospitalisation and confinement. You will want to be there as much as possible, yet you cannot become a slave to your own imagination about what you should or should not do. Very few people are so free from obligations that they can live in the hospital with the patient. All you can do is your best. Do not expect more of yourself.

Other people besides the patient need you. Your work needs you. You need you. Do not let a tyrannical sense of martyrdom obsess you. Do all that you possibly can, and let others help. If you have a home church, tell your pastor about your needs and limitations.

The patient may not feel like having a constant stream of visitors, anyway. That might be tiring. Ask the patient how he feels about visitors. It may be that he would like some time alone. On the other hand, too little visiting can make the patient feel abandoned, alone, and very depressed.

It is so hard to know what to say during a visit. What should a visitor say or not say when visiting a cancer

patient in the hospital? Making conversation is sometimes extremely difficult, especially if the patient is depressed and anxious. You know that he does not want to talk about the weather any more than you do.

Here are some suggestions, however:

Do not tell the patient how "lucky" he is. He does not feel one bit lucky.

Do not tell him how great he looks, unless he really does. You can pick out something that actually does look good, for example, Your colour looks much better today, or, You look like you had a good night's rest.

Super-happy and bouncy visitors may make the patient feel worse. Take it easy until you see how he is feeling.

Do not tell him what a rough week you have had.

Do not tell him that you know just how he feels. You do not.

Do ask him if he feels like talking. Be an active listener. Encourage him to express himself to you.

He might like you to read to him some words of comfort from the Bible. Paul wrote the book of Philippians while in prison, yet the book is overflowing with joy. That might be a good place to read.

Go into the room with a warm smile and say hi. A hug or pat on the arm can express much of what you want to say. You can find out what is on the patient's mind by saying something like, How are you coping?

The sense of touch is extremely important, especially when a person is in the midst of trauma. Very often people recoil from the cancer patient, standing back from the bed, refusing to touch him, giving the impression that the diagnosis might be leprosy. *Cancer is not contagious.* Hold the patient's hand and sit on the side of the bed if it is comfortable for him. Your physical closeness will be solacing.

What kind of emotional responses might the cancer patient have? One of the greatest problems of family members is dealing with the emotional upset of the cancer patient when they are also traumatised.

You might as well expect the cancer patient to exhibit any or all of these emotional responses: anger, fear, depression, irritability, sleeplessness, and bizarre dreams. Increased sexual feelings often are part of unusual tension and stress, and the patient may feel guilty because of these feelings. If he or she does not know how to handle guilt, that will add to the anxiety.

A special problem for men experiencing the progressively debilitating process of terminal cancer is the sense of a "loss of manliness". This problem causes depression, which may be expressed in hostility toward the family, especially the wife.

What special problems face the family when the condition is terminal and in the last stages and the patient is being cared for at home? About 30 per cent of patients are cared for at home and families who choose to care for a terminally ill patient at home usually are glad afterwards that they have done so. It is a stressful time, but many families grow very close and find unforeseen blessings in such a situation. A useful book on this subject is *Life Before Death* by Ann Cartwright, published in 1973 by Routledge & Kegan Paul.

The word *terminal* sometimes suggests to people that nothing more can be done for the patient. This is not true. It may be that nothing more can be done to cure the cancer, but there is always much that can be done to make the patient more comfortable.

The primary caretaker will not be able to manage all the bedside nursing responsibilities. Bathing, feeding, changing dressings, changing sheets, changing the patient's position, relieving constipation, and sitting up at night are just a few of the many important things to be done. Frequent rubdowns of back, buttocks, elbows, heels, and knees also make the patient more comfortable. A comfortable, dry bed is as essential as loving, compassionate nursing care. If you are not the primary caretaker, offer to help in any way you can.

About half of the people who die from cancer experience no pain at all from the disease, and powerful pain medication is available for those who do. Visiting nurses can sometimes come to your home and help you with specific problems regarding pain, feeding, and so forth.

Most families in this situation need some sort of special equipment—hospital beds, walkers, wheelchairs. This kind of equipment is usually available from a number of sources. Your GP will be able to give you details, or ring the Social Services (the telephone number will be in your local telephone directory), the British Red Cross (9 Grosvenor Crescent, London, SW1), the Liza Sainsbury Foundation (8/10 Crown Hill, Croydon, Surrey, CR0 1RY), or one of the hospices. Your GP can also advise you as to the availability of visiting nurses such as the District Nurses, or Macmillan Nurses (through the National Society for Cancer Relief, Anchor House, 15 Britten Street, London, SW3). The Marie Curie Foundation offers a free night-nurse service (28 Belgrave Square, London, SW1), and the Social Services also provide nursing support.

Inability to sleep is another commonly encountered problem for family members, and this problem adds to the emotional stress of the situation. The ability to cope is directly related to being rested. *You must get adequate sleep.*

Trying to maintain normal family activities during a time such as this is nearly impossible. Ask for help. If you are an extremely capable person, members of the extended family may not know that you need help. Explain your needs specifically. If you do not have an extended family, your church family will help if the pastor is made aware of your needs.

I find that I am depending on our doctor for emotional support and am usually disappointed. What should I

expect from him? Family members and the patient tend to look to the doctor for emotional support on an ongoing basis, particularly in the last stages. Most people express the desire for the doctor to give more emotional support and to take more time to explain what is happening. Some doctors give this kind of emotional support, and some do not.

Families and patients often endow the doctor with superhuman qualities, then are disappointed to find that he is only human. Most doctors working with cancer patients are extremely knowledgeable and concerned. But they are just human beings with limited knowledge doing the best they can. It is really not fair to expect them to be more than that.

What about financial problems? Cancer costs can be overwhelming, but there is a variety of financial help available for the cancer sufferer and his family. The benefits available through the Social Services range widely, from help with prescriptions to the installation of necessary equipment within the patient's home.

It is also worth approaching any of the many cancer charities for financial help, for example, the National Society for Cancer Relief and the Malcolm Sargent Cancer Fund For Children (14 Abingdon Road, London W8). The Leukaemia Care Society offers emotional and financial assistance, and also arranges holidays for child sufferers (write to PO Box 82, Exeter, Devon, EX2 5DP). Emergency financial help is available through the Marie Curie Foundation.

SPIRITUAL NEEDS OF A CANCER PATIENT

Family members are primarily concerned about the physical needs of the cancer patient: the treatments, procedures, chemotherapy protocol. These needs are important. His physical comfort is, of course, one of the main concerns. Emotional needs are also recognised. The cancer patient needs emotional support in dealing with circumstances that may be, for the first time in his life, totally beyond his control. Spiritual needs, however, are rarely recognised. Hospital chaplains visit the patients routinely, but often even they do not recognise spiritual needs.

Spiritual needs have symptoms as do physical and emotional needs. We are responsible for being aware of and sensitive to those needs as well.

Nell Collins, the cancer missionary, conducts a seminar for nurses on the subject "How to Recognise a Spiritual Need." The following are the most easily recognised symptoms.

Rejection of people. Often a patient will turn his face to the wall and refuse to communicate with anybody. Sometimes this is because his visitor refuses to talk about spiritual matters, and the patient does not want to talk about anything else.

Tears. Be sensitive to the patient's need to cry. In our culture, men often feel that they should not shed tears, so you may help by saying, It sometimes helps just to have a good cry. Though tears can be a sign of many other feelings, such as worry, anxiety, or loneliness, it is possible the patient is distraught because he feels he does not have the right relationship with God.

Floor-pacing. This person is often quite sleepy but cannot sleep because he has a spiritual need that is not being met. So he paces the floor.

Change in normal sleep patterns. A spiritual need could be expressed by a radical change in sleep patterns. Either inability to sleep (insomnia) or sleeping far more than normal is a danger signal.

Open admission of fear. If a patient says, I'm afraid, give him a chance to express his fears; let him talk about them. Ask him, *What* are you afraid of? not, *Why* are you afraid?

Despondency. The dumps. No matter how much wealth or success has been realised in life, a person will be unutterably sad until he has had his spiritual needs met. Only eternal confidence brings comfort in human distress.

Egocentric trip. The only person this patient can talk about is himself. The pronouns *I, me,* and *my* are prominent in his conversation. We tend to turn away from this person, but he may be self-centred because of an unmet spiritual need. Let him talk, and listen sensitively for the heartache that he so desperately wants and needs to express.

Spiritual introversion. This person refuses to talk to his church leader or anyone else about spiritual matters. A spiritual withdrawing often looks as if the patient does not want to discuss these things; frequently the reverse is true.

Once the spiritual needs have been recognised, then you can begin to help the patient. But first, make sure that you yourself are not confused about death, what it means, and possibly even your own relationship with God. If you are not sure of your own beliefs, you should direct the patient to some other person who can help. Ask if he wants a visit from the pastor of a Bible-believing church.

Next, *listen* to him. This is probably the most helpful thing you can do. The cancer patient will be frustrated if you will not let him talk about his fears. Even if the prognosis is good, he may want to talk about the possibility of death. Let him talk, and do not be patronising ("Now, now, you don't need to be worrying about *that*"). If the prognosis is poor, the family may be so concerned with, How are we going to tell him? that they fail to hear when the patient tells *them* that he is dying.

Let the patient talk about death if he wants to. If you cringe and refuse to talk, or if you change the subject every time he mentions it, you might as well be saying, It's too horrible to even suggest. That attitude is not helpful.

Megan Hudson, a twenty-two-year-old girl with para-thyroid cancer, writes:

> What I craved above all else was the opportunity to talk about my fears, but listening seemed to be difficult for many people. They seemed compelled to minimise the risks, to be optimistic. Perhaps quiet listening was too passive, too easy, and they had to be active to "fix things up". But reassuring statistics weren't reassuring, and being told not to worry was no comfort. I wanted sympathy and commiseration, not cheering up. "What a hard time you're going through," not, "Everything will be all right."[1]

Remember, hope is vitally important. The patient should have hope, but not false hope. Promoters of quack cures can cheat cancer patients out of millions of dollars a year because they do not sell cures, they sell hope—false hope.

There is also a difference between temporary hope and ultimate hope. The patient should know that difference. It is good to hope that the chemotherapy will work, to hope that the radiotherapy will be effective, to hope that the third surgery will take care of the cancer. It is also good to hope that research will find a new cure for the kind of cancer he has.

Do not take this temporary hope away from the patient. Many patients, including those who are true believers, maintain to the very end some kind of hope that the physical condition will improve. The patient should not be made to feel that he has been "given up".

On the other hand, the family should be sensitive to the fact that the patient's hopes will change as he begins accepting the reality of his situation. It will only frustrate the patient for you to keep talking about hopes he recognises to be no longer valid. This is a time for real communication among family members—not for pretending and play-acting. Sometimes families invent an elaborate network of deception to "protect" the patient from the truth. The deception forces the patient to bear his fears and anxieties *all alone*; ultimately, it is a cruel thing to do.

Temporary hope is hope in the things of this world. Ultimate hope is hope in God. It is ultimate hope that will give peace.

6

IF CANCER STRIKES A CHILD

Kevin Jones just had his eighth birthday party with balloons, party hats, and a cake with a football player on top. (Kevin is crazy about Arsenal.) Just another birthday party, you say?

Kevin's mum cried inside when he blew out all his candles, and his dad blinked back the tears. His older sister had to leave the table. They all knew that this was a very special birthday. Every birthday for Kevin is special.

Kevin is a boy with acute lymphocytic leukaemia. It has been two years since his diagnosis, and he is in remission and doing well. He is a victim of childhood cancer, but he goes to school, is a Cub Scout, takes piano lessons, and wants to be a doctor when he grows up.

He is planning on growing up.

When the diagnosis of Kevin's cancer was made, his parents were horrified. They had always thought of cancer as something an older person might get, since it becomes more common with increasing age. But a child! In an address delivered in Marseilles, France, December 1977, C. Everett Koop, MD, then Surgeon-in-Chief of the Children's Hospital of Philadelphia, stated, "The diagnosis of cancer in a child is not only difficult to believe; it is unthinkable."

In the 1950s, victims of childhood leukaemia and other cancers were given little hope. The main concern, then, was to make the child as comfortable as possible during his last weeks or months.

While no absolute cure has yet been found, and cancer is second only to accidents as a cause of death in childhood, medical science has made great advances in the treatment of these diseases. By combining surgery, radiotherapy, and multi-drug chemotherapy in a programme designed for the individual patient, more and more victims of childhood cancer can hope for full recovery.

These hopes indeed give comfort to the child and the family, but at the same time the months and even years of intense treatment cause the entire family unit to experience great stress. Death is still a real enemy, and the war against that enemy is often painful, usually financially staggering, and always emotionally draining. The spectre of death is always looming because, as Dr Koop added, "In spite of the major therapeutic advances that have been made in the management of solid tumours and leukaemia to the end that the mortality is considerably improved, more children still die of cancer than are cured of it."

PARENTS IN EMOTIONAL SHOCK

Most people do not know the great advances that have been made in the last several years in treating childhood cancer. Initially, when the diagnosis is made, the parents are just overwhelmed. They think that childhood cancer always means death, and they go into a state of emotional shock.

Andy McCord is a lively two-year-old who likes *Sesame Street* and building blocks. To look at him, you would never know he had ever been sick.

Andy was diagnosed with neuroblastoma when four months old. This particular kind of cancer is of the primitive nerve cells and usually first appears in the abdomen. Andy's tumour was wrapped around his aorta, the major vessel from his heart.

"They gave us very little hope that he'd even survive surgery," says Mrs McCord. "My husband and I went into a kind of shock. You can't believe the horror of being told your child has cancer. It's just beyond belief how terrible it is."

Little Andy came through the surgery successfully, then was started on radiation and chemotherapy. He was quite sick during the time of treatment, and the McCords went numbly through those weeks, too scared even to pray.

During that time they began to see the need for a source of strength beyond themselves. "I believe that God began to bring Christian friends to us," says Mrs McCord, "and they helped us understand how Christ could be the answer to our every need. Now we depend totally on him, no matter what it is that we are facing. We just don't know what we'd do without Christ in our lives."

RELATED PROBLEMS

The Hospital for Sick Children, Great Ormond Street in London is, among other things, a treatment centre for childhood cancer. The staff of the department of haematology and oncology make a serious effort to help families and cancer patients face certain problems and circumstances that often accompany the treatment of childhood cancer.

Guilt in parents. The first emotional response seen in the parents is an enormous sense of guilt. Penelope Brock, MD, Leukaemia Research Fellow at Great Ormond Street, stated in an interview: "Without exception, every parent when told that their child has cancer, tortures themselves with ideas of what they could have done to prevent it happening. Some put the blame directly on to themselves, others put it on the doctor or other medical personnel who 'took too long' to make the diagnosis. The early symptoms of cancer are frequently vague and resemble other childhood illnesses. The child has often been treated initially for an infection before the underlying cause is discovered. However, the reason why children get cancer is as yet unknown, so there is nothing that any parent could have done to prevent his child acquiring it. There is therefore nothing to feel guilty about, angry perhaps.''

Another kind of guilt revolves around the parent-child relationship. Under stress, any parent will probably feel guilty about past failures, both real and imagined. The diagnosis of cancer in the child magnifies the sense of guilt. This sense of being personally responsible for the child's illness can be all-encompassing.

Overprotection. Parents of a child with cancer will inevitably be overprotective. When the parents know their child has an illness that may take his life, the natural human reaction is to try to protect that child from any further harm. The result, unhappily, is a life that is anything but normal. Decisions about activity must be made on an individual basis, but in general the child should go back to school as soon as he is able. He should play with other children. Brothers and sisters should be allowed to have friends over to visit. The parents should feel free to leave him with a baby-sitter. Family vacations and holidays abroad should not be discontinued if the child is doing well.

Of course, parents need to be sensitive to real dangers. Most children with cancer should not be exposed to certain illnesses, such as chicken pox, and they need to stay home from school when exposure is a possibility.

Negative response of others. Parents need to be warned that other relatives and family friends may have surprisingly negative reactions. For example, one parent found that her baby-sitter would no longer stay with the children, and some friends refused to come into the house. Even though cancer is not contagious, some people think it is. The parents suddenly have to deal with other people's fears as well as their own.

Parents may need to go to the child's school and explain the disease, the treatment, and the side effects, so the children and teachers will be able to treat the child as normally as possible.

One of my daughter's school friends is almost a celebrity in her fifth grade classroom because of her leukaemia. She has given the class much information concerning the disease, and one day she gave a talk on bone marrow aspirations. This kind of communication is helpful in bringing about understanding and normal relationships with the other children and teachers.

Need for professional care. Parents are often overwhelmed by a sense of being incapable of caring for their child. Penelope Brock, MD at Great Ormond Street Hospital for Sick Children says, "Staff members need to be sensitive to the fact that the parents have always taken care of this child. Now, suddenly, all these other people are taking care of him, and the parent doesn't know how to do some of the things that need to be done. We try to teach the parents to participate in the care of the child. It is comforting to the child, and the parents don't feel left out."

Frightening experiences. Children who are diagnosed with cancer are suddenly faced with many new experiences: frightened parents, serious-faced strangers, a hospital bed, tubes, machines, equipment, and needles. He must face procedures and treatments that either hurt or make him nauseated. Usually the child has never been seriously ill before. He is scared.

Change in body image. The child and the parents should be prepared for a possible change in body image. Very often children under treatment for cancer lose their hair, and frequently the chemotherapy causes a puffiness of the face and abdomen. They should know in advance that these changes might take place, but that the hair should grow back, and the puffiness should go away.

Complications. The child with leukaemia or other forms of childhood cancer always risks developing serious complications from the therapy. The treatment for the disease may go very well, but other problems, such as haemorrhage or infection, may arise and become very grave.

DISCIPLINE

Many family problems arise normally in the area of discipline, and if a child has a life-threatening disease, the difficulties multiply.

Often a father and mother will disagree about when, if, and how to discipline. This situation leads to division and strife, and if it is compounded by the knowledge that a child has cancer, the family relationships all suffer. The parents must communicate with each other, decide what behaviour is reasonable to expect, then support each other in carrying it out.

Though life will never be the same once cancer has been diagnosed, it is important that the family return to "normal" as soon as possible.

Part of treating a child "normally" involves the area of discipline. Many parents become extremely lax, and that is not healthy for the child.

Every child, even a sick child, needs limits set and enforced. A child's being sick does not mean he will no longer be wilful, disobedient, or rebellious. Any child, sick or not, will test the limits to see if they will be enforced. For the child's sense of security, it is important to set reasonable limits and then make certain that he is lovingly kept within those limits.

In setting limits, however, the parents need to be flexible enough to adjust to changing situations. The treatment for cancer is often painful and stress-producing. The child is undergoing treatments that may cause his behaviour to change. He may respond to the treatments with anger, resentment, bitterness, and jealousy of those who are well. These negative emotions, in turn, can cause unacceptable behaviour.

The parent needs to be understanding and kind. The child will not understand these powerful negative emotions and will feel guilty about having them. He may not even be able to identify them. The parent must help him understand why he feels the way he does, perhaps by expressing in words what the child is feeling. ("You are feeling angry because you want to be well. You wish you could be well again.")

The parent can help a child express his negative emotions in this manner. Often a torrent of emotions will then pour out, like water from a crumbling dam. Allow the child to express himself. Do not be shocked at his feelings. These feelings need to be expressed, and a sensitive parent can be of tremendous help to a child in this area.

TRUTH

Children who are old enough to understand must be told the truth about their disease. One of the most difficult times for the parents is telling the child that he has cancer or leukaemia, but it is vital that those words be used, even with very young children. If you try to hide the truth from the child, he will not be able to come to terms with his illness; he will fantasise about what is wrong.

If you do not tell him, he will find out sooner or later, and his trust in you will be damaged. Usually hospital staff members help parents over this hurdle by using the words in a matter-of-fact manner during treatment at the time of diagnosis.

How the truth is told is important. For example, when one six-year-old was diagnosed with non-Hodgkins lymphoma, the conversation went something like this:

Dr A.: "Do you know why you are here, Robert?"

Robert: "No."

Dr A.: "Would you like to know what's wrong with you?"

Robert: "Yes."

Dr A.: "Robert, you have a disease called *cancer*. Have you ever known anyone who had cancer?"

Robert: "No."

Dr A.: "Your body is made up of many cells. When you cut yourself or hurt yourself, the cells may be injured, so some body cells divide to repair the injury. However, with cancer, the cells divide without a need, and then you have extra cells. So we will give you treatments to try to stop the cells from dividing. [Dr A. then drew a diagram to show Robert how the cells divide.] Sometimes people are frightened of cancer because they have heard of people who died from cancer, but you don't need to be afraid, because we will try to make you better."

Truth can be brutal, but it does not need to be. Give the child the facts in a loving, gentle way. Many questions will come up during the course of treatment, and all his questions should be answered as simply and honestly as possible. It is not necessary to dwell on the fact of the illness either and to talk about it all the time. To do so would make a miserable and far-from-normal situation.

Most school-age children are very interested in the nature of their disease. An excellent book for children with leukaemia is *Jenny has Leukaemia* by Anne Nicholson and

Janice Thompson, which is available free through the Malcolm Sargent Cancer Fund. Another excellent book written for children, but extremely informative for parents too, is *You and Leukemia: a Day at a Time* by Lynn S. Baker. This is an American book, which can be obtained through BACUP (121/123 Charterhouse Street, London, EC1M 6AA), who also provide a leaflet called *Coping with Childhood Leukaemia* by Nancy Hallett.

If the time should come that your child's prognosis is poor, you must share that with him. Do not take away all hope for finding a medicine that might help, but acknowledge that he may not be able to get well. He probably knows anyway, but if you can talk about it, he will not have to bear this knowledge alone.

A mother told me that one of her most meaningful memories was of the day she told her teenage son that he might not recover from his leukaemia.

"Do you mean that I'm going to die?" he asked her.

"I don't know the answer to that, son. But it is possible."

Then they both cried.

Later he told her, "Thanks, Mum. It's good to have someone to cry with."

Because mother and son were able to have that very difficult conversation, the way was opened for them to talk freely about heaven and the reality of a special place being prepared there for all who place their faith in Christ. During his last days, they talked almost constantly about his loving Saviour who would be with him eternally.

I cried when I read Mikie Sherman's account of the death of her daughter in *The Leukemic Child*.[1] Elizabeth died at age seven, after two-and-a-half years of treatment. I cried because Mrs Sherman never was able to talk about death with Elizabeth. She discussed the fact that professionals disagree about whether or not a child should be shielded from death. Some psychologists and psychiatrists believe that children should be "protected" from the harsh reality of dying. Other professionals, however, disagree, maintaining that children can cope with truth far better than with playacting.

My heart grieved for Mrs Sherman and her daughter when she said, "I had no heaven nor personal God to offer Elizabeth." How tragic.

I believe that all young children who die are safe in God's loving care, but I am so sorry that Mrs Sherman and Elizabeth went through that dreadful time without his comfort.

Children of different ages have varying kinds of fears about death. The preschooler may not understand the finality of death, but the school-age child will. Most youngsters are open, honest, and eager to have specific information about what heaven might be like.

A fear common to many children stems from associating death with the word *sleep*. Perhaps when his grandfather died, the child was told, Grandpa is sleeping. He also may have heard of someone dying in his sleep. Because of that, the child may be afraid to sleep or afraid for you to sleep. Discuss with him the use of the word *sleep* and assure him that it is safe to sleep.

A great fear concerning death is the fear of separation from loved ones. Emphasise to the child that Jesus is his very best friend, and he will be with him always, no matter what happens. This truth will help the child deal with his greatest fear: fear of the unknown.

GUILT IN CHILDREN

Sometimes a child fears he has done something bad that caused the cancer. One little boy had heard on television that smoking causes cancer. He was convinced that he had the disease because he had sneaked a couple of his father's cigarettes and smoked them. He may feel he is being "punished" for other times he has misbehaved. Children with cancer need to know that they are not being punished for being bad. But they should also know that God has provided a way for total forgiveness through trust in Jesus Christ.

SIBLINGS

A child with cancer usually has brothers and/or sisters. These children, too, need information to help them deal with this situation.

Because of the nature of the disease, childhood cancer is usually a long-term problem, having both crisis times and back-to-normal times. Both younger children and older children need to know what is happening. If they are not told that Johnny has a serious problem, they will not understand why he is getting so much attention. They need to be assured that mummy and daddy love them just as much as they do Johnny, and the parents need to be made aware of the fact that the siblings need love and attention, too.

A small child needs to be told the truth, gently and sensitively, in language he can understand.

Perhaps he could be told something like this (with the information adjusted to fit the situation): "Johnny has something seriously wrong with his blood. It is called leukaemia. This can be a very dangerous disease, and children sometimes die from it. We expect Johnny will live for a long, long time, but we must do everything we can to help him.

"Johnny will be receiving treatment at the hospital. This is very important to help him get better. Sometimes he will be very sick, and sometimes he will feel just fine. He will be getting a lot of attention. We want you to know that we love you just as much as Johnny, even though we might have to spend a lot more time with him for a while."

If the prognosis becomes very poor, and death draws

near, the siblings should know ahead of time so that they are not caught unprepared for it. The Christian parent can express the reality of the situation, yet give real comfort and hope. The parent might say, "You know, dear, that Johnny has been very ill. He has been taking medicine all this time to help him get well. Sometimes medicine works, and sometimes it doesn't. If Johnny's medicine doesn't work, he might go to be with Jesus sooner than we had thought. If the medicine does work, he'll be with us a long, long time. Right now we just can't know for sure what is going to happen. But we can trust God that if Johnny does go to be with Jesus, he will be happy there, and he won't ever hurt again."

Children are truly amazing in the way they rally when the truth is made clear. A brother or sister of a leukaemia victim might willingly, even eagerly, go through the pain and trauma of being the donor for a bone marrow transplant. This relatively new procedure is becoming more and more successful as problems are worked out, though it is done in only a few hospitals. The point is that the other children in the family want and need to be included, even if not in such a dramatic way as donating bone marrow. Give your children the opportunity to be part of the family in a meaningful way during this difficult time.

If death should occur, I believe that both younger and older siblings should be allowed to attend funeral services. The funeral provides the opportunity to see that the loved one is dead and is not coming back. The funeral service gives all loved ones a way to work through their grief and accept the reality of death.

FACING DEATH TWICE

In the address mentioned earlier, Dr Koop says: "When death finally comes, there is a sense of release for the hospital staff, the community, and for the family. The family who loses a child with cancer really loses him twice. They lose him first when they finally come to the realisation that he has a hopeless diagnosis and a hopeless prognosis. They lose him the second time when physical death overtakes him. In a sense, the first death is more difficult, and the second provides some feeling of relief. It should be said in passing that even when the cancer patient recovers and eventually is called 'cured', the family, wondering about the prognosis, goes through all of the same agonising months that are experienced by those who eventually lose their child."

RELINQUISHMENT

To be freed from the bondage of worry, the Christian parent at one time or another must come to the place where, as an act of the will, he literally surrenders his child into God's perfect and sovereign care. For some spiritually mature parents, this relinquishment might come early, perhaps when the child is born. For others, this act of giving the child to God occurs at a time of critical illness. For most, the act of relinquishment will have to be repeated, because fear and worry can cause a parent to "take back" what he has given to the Lord.

In any case, relinquishment is one of the most difficult jobs of a parent. But it is *absolutely essential* if the parent is to have any peace in life.

"It was sheer agony," said Marie Logan, the mother of a one-year-old little girl with neuroblastoma, "just standing by and watching my baby suffer. It was almost like a dream—no, a nightmare—to think this could happen to our only little girl.

"I didn't want to cry in front of her, so I'd have to leave the room sometimes, just to cry. Our hospital has a room where people can go to be alone, so one day I went there to pray.

" 'God', I said, 'you know how dearly I love this baby. I just can't bear the thought of her being taken from me. But I know that she really belongs to you. She is your child. You've just given us the privilege of taking care of her for a while. I thank you for that. I don't know what is going to happen with her, but all I can do is trust you. She's your child, and I know you love her even more than I do. So today, I put her totally in your hands, and I will trust you to do whatever you see is best in her life.'

"It was so amazing", Mrs Logan continues, "the peace that God granted to me at that moment. It was like I'd been released from chains. I went back upstairs and found my little girl sleeping peacefully.

"She is still a very sick little girl. The doctors are saying her condition is poor. I know she might not get well. But she is God's child, and he knows what is best. Even though it is hard, we can rest in that."

How many more birthdays will these little children have? No one knows. But then, none of us knows how many days or years we have to live. In any case, it is not advisable to move up a birthday party a few months because death appears imminent. Do not celebrate Christmas in October. Doing so has been found to be devastating for the child, the parents, and anyone else involved.

"Children are killed every day in automobile accidents," says one mother. "We can't spend the time we have together worrying about when it will end. Life is too precious. We simply have to live while we can, for all of our sakes. I know that my child has cancer, and I know that he may die from it. But we're going to live from day to day. That makes every day very special."

7

IS GOD ALWAYS GOOD?

Anne Jones, mother of a six-year-old boy, was thirty-two when she discovered a lump in her breast. The biopsy proved the tumour to be malignant, and she immediately had a radical mastectomy of the left side.

"I tried to be really brave at first," she says. "I was going to show everyone how beautifully I could cope—I'd be the model example of courage. I was going to fly through this thing with no problem, just like a breeze.

"I was able to muddle through for a little while before I fell apart. Completely. I just went to pieces, got hysterical, and my fury with God just poured out.

"I denied that there could possibly be a God who would make anyone suffer the anguish I was suffering. I was very bitter; my pride was hurt. I wanted another child and they wouldn't let me get pregnant again. I even had to go in and have my tubes tied. I was so miserable, and I was going to make everyone just as miserable as I was.

"I shook my fist at God and screamed down the hall, 'How *dare* you do this to me. How dare you!' There just could not be a God, let alone that 'good God' I had always heard about, who could do something like this to me.

"I saw myself as ugly, deformed. I thought that everyone saw my ugliness. When they looked at me, I was sure that was all they saw. I struck out at everyone and everything. I hated everybody. I struck out in words, in viciousness, in bitterness, with a scowl on my face. I was going to make everyone else feel just as miserable as I did."

Anne was caught up in the middle of tragedy. Faced with cancer, Anne found she had to know more about God. Though she was furious with what was happening in her life, she knew that she was bewildered about God and his character.

IS GOD GOOD?

Is God really good? Or is he vicious and malicious?

It is easy to become confused about the nature of God. Some feel we tend to see God the way we view our earthly fathers. Those of us who are blessed with good earthly fathers, though they are not perfect, have a far easier time seeing God as he truly is.

Though everyone is a creation of God, a person becomes his child by accepting Jesus Christ as Saviour. When that decision is made, a person is born into God's family. What a wonderful thing it is to be able to call the God of the universe "Father".

As God, however, he is a good and perfect father—and this is where we sometimes run into problems. We all have ideas as to what a good father is like. We know that a good father is fair, kind, just, loving, and forgiving. We know that a good father helps his children when they are in need. We know that a good father disciplines his children; he does not let them run wild. We know that a good father takes time to care for and be interested in the daily lives of his children.

Earthly fathers, however, fall short of this ideal. Our concept of God can be affected by an earthly father who is angry, vengeful, and unforgiving. A weak and ineffectual father, or a father who is too busy for his child, can distort in a person's mind the character of the perfect and sovereign Creator of the universe.

Can we imagine perfection? Can we understand sovereignty? Probably not. Our finite minds are limited, but God is not.

The Scriptures declare God to be the supreme ruler. Lewis Sperry Chafer says in *Major Bible Themes*:

> The attributes of God make clear that God is supreme over all. He yields to no other power, authority, or glory, and is not subject to any absolute greater than Himself. He represents perfection to an infinite degree in every aspect of His being. He can never be surprised, defeated, or uncertain. However, without sacrificing His authority or jeopardising the final realisation of His perfect will, it has pleased God to give men a measure of freedom of choice, and for the exercise of this choice God holds man responsible.[1]

Because God is sovereign, the blessed Controller of all things, we can know that nothing beyond his scope of power can touch our lives. Every detail of our lives is within his command.

At the same time, God is love.

Merrill Unger defines *love* as "the highest characteristic of God, the one attribute in which all others harmoniously blend. The love of God is more than kindness or benevolence. The latter may be exercised toward irrational creatures, but love is directed toward rational, personal beings."[2]

WHY TRAGEDY?

But Anne Jones asked a valid question. If God is so good and loves us so much, then *why* does he allow tragedy to enter our lives? How can a good God do a rotten thing like this?

To deal with this question, we have to go back a long, long way—to the beginning.

The first chapters of the Bible tell of beginnings: the beginning of the universe, of plant and animal life, of human life, and of our problems in the world. Though these chapters have been hotly debated, they still stand as the only reasonable explanation for why we have trouble in this world.

If a person can accept what is stated in these chapters, he has gone a long way toward understanding why we have tragedy, disease, death, and unhappiness on this planet earth. No one says the Genesis account gives a complete, detailed report of everything that transpired in those days, but it does tell of an all-powerful Creator. This omnipotent One but spoke and brought from nothing our planet and solar system. The billions of other stars and planets, across space so vast we cannot begin to comprehend it, appeared at his word. From the infinite reaches of outer space to the microscopic world of the individual cell, God created it all.

THE CREATOR LOVES US

After all of that, the most amazing report in Genesis is that this Creator of everything loves and cares for us individually. He knows about and cares about the tiniest happening in this physical universe. He knows how many hairs are on each of our heads; he knows when a sparrow falls from a tree. From the very first, he has cared for and loved each one of us. Personally. Individually. One-to-one.

God did not want us to experience disease and death. He created a flawless world. The rosebushes had no thorns. The perfect amount of moisture caressed the vibrant blossoms and lush greenery. The sky and streams had no pollution.

God created man, as the Bible says, "in his own image," his character and being a reflection of the Creator. Man's human body was made from the dust of the earth, but his spiritual nature was "breathed in" by God himself. No animal has this spiritual nature, or God-consciousness.

Adam's and Eve's created bodies never had a pimple, never had a wrinkle. Certainly they never had cancer.

God's creation was perfect. So what happened?

ORIGIN OF SUFFERING

The first couple, created by God, was in a state of moral purity. This purity was necessary in order for them to have fellowship with God, who is absolute holiness. Because of the holiness of his divine character, he must, in the most complete sense, be separated from evil.

Along with moral purity, Adam and Eve had freedom of choice. God could have made them in such a way that sinning would have been impossible, but he wanted them to be free to choose to love him.

God created man for his glory and to have fellowship with him, but man chose to go his own way. The first man and woman rebelled against God in the matter of eating from a certain tree in the Garden. This act seems a small infraction to us, but it demonstrates the seriousness of sin. That sin caused a great gulf between man and his Creator, and God's perfect planet was no longer perfect.

That long-ago choice was a turning point in human history, and the results were catastrophic. Disease, death, and hardship became facts of life on this earth. The inclination to go against God was passed down from generation to generation.

Our rosebushes have thorns; we have cancer. Our bodies deteriorate, and we need bifocals. We have heart attacks and heartaches. "The whole creation groaneth and travaileth in pain" (Rom. 8:22).

In spite of the tragedy that sin brought to the earth in terms of human suffering, God's love was so great that he immediately set in motion his plan to redeem lost humanity.

Through all the centuries, both before and after Calvary, God remains the blessed Controller of all things, tenderly, lovingly drawing us to himself. Though at times it may seem he has forsaken us on this sin-scarred earth and has left us alone in our miseries, he has not.

God does not always let us know why specific tragedies happen: why a seventeen-year-old boy should lose his arm to bone cancer, why a man in the prime of life should succumb to lung cancer, why a young wife and mother should lose her breast.

The Bible, however, gives us much evidence that problems and trials are part of life on this planet. We are, as Eliphaz told Job, "born unto trouble, as the sparks fly upward" (Job 5:7).

Jesus confirmed this with probably the greatest understatement of all time: "In the world ye shall have tribulation" (John 16:33).

But God does not leave us alone in the midst of sorrow and despair. Because of his great love for us, he has provided a way for us to reach him—a way, not *out* of all stressful times, but *through* them.

8

THE ULTIMATE HOPE

What hope is there for the cancer patient? Every cancer patient hopes for full recovery, and for many these hopes will be fulfilled. Medical science has made great strides in cancer research. As previously mentioned, the cancer patient before this century had almost no hope of recovery. Death was inevitable. Today, as more and more effective treatments are developed, more cancer patients than ever can hope for complete recovery.

For some, however, the hope for full restoration is illusive. These patients intuitively start changing their hopes: Alice now hopes she can live long enough to see her children graduate from high school; Jim hopes to see his son take over the business. "If I can just see my daughter get married," says Barbara.

But if these hopes also fade, what hope is left for the cancer patient whose hope of physical recovery seems dim at best?

HOPE IS MEDICINAL

Hope is vital.

S. I. McMillen, MD, tells about the profound meaning of hope in his book *None of These Diseases*. He illustrates with verse how different people react to the same stressful circumstances.

> Two men look out through the same bars:
> One sees the mud, and one the stars.
>   Frederick Langbridge

Many of some 31,000 Allied soldiers imprisoned in Japan and Korea in the 1940s couldn't see anything except mud. Dr Harold Wolff states that even though these prisoners were offered enough food, "the prisoner became apathetic, listless, neither ate nor drank, helped himself in no way, stared into space and finally died." Of the 31,000 imprisoned, over 8,000 died. Dr Wolff states that many of these deaths were caused by "despair and deprivation of human support and affection". Dr Wolff, who is editor-in-chief of *Archives and* [sic] *Neurology and Psychiatry*, declares that "Hope, like faith and a purpose in life, is medicinal. This is not merely a statement of belief, but a conclusion proved by meticulously controlled scientific experiment."[1]

Scientists now know that we cannot live without hope. But what is this rather nebulous quality that is so important to our very existence? The dictionary calls *hope* "confident trust". The question is, Confident trust in what? In what has the cancer patient placed his hope?

Does he hope that the surgeon removed all of the cancer cells? Of course. Does he hope the radiotherapy will prevent the return of the disease? Certainly. Does he hope the chemotherapy will stop its spread, or that he will achieve a remission? The answer is obvious—every cancer patient and his family hope that these measures will be effective. He may be hoping that research will find a new cure for the cancer facing him. It is good to have these hopes.

The problem is that these hopes, good as they are, can be disappointing. They are temporary hopes, that is, hopes in the things of this world. These hopes may become evasive, illusive, and often totally shattered. If we have placed *all* our hope in medical science, we may be bitterly disappointed. There is a vast difference between human hope, which is based on the things around us, and eternal hope, which is based on God and what he tells us in his Word. Because God has revealed himself to us through Scripture, we can know him in a personal way and be confident concerning a future that might, in an earthly sense, seem bleak.

REAL HOPE

Douglas Evans is a man who found himself in the situation of discovering his hope shattered. A great believer in man's scientific ability to cure disease, he rested totally on this hope when he found that he had cancer. When he began to see how disappointing earthly hopes can be, he called Nell Collins.

Douglas looked out the window by his hospital bed. Tears welled up in his eyes; he bit his lip, trying to stop the flow.

"Go ahead," Nell said. "It's OK to cry."

He wiped his eyes and blew his nose.

"Funny," he said, "I wasn't half so scared the first time." (The first time was two years ago when he had surgery for a bowel obstruction.)

"I wasn't too surprised to find out it was cancer," he said. "I'd been having some pain and unusual bleeding. The surgery was no fun, of course. And I hated the prospect of wearing a colostomy bag. But for some reason, that time the cancer itself didn't really worry me too much. The doctors kept saying that they thought I'd be all right. My wife was wonderful about it. She just laughed and called the colostomy bag my 'porta-potty'. But now—"

Nell had known Douglas since his first surgery. She had been asked to visit him by one of his wife's friends. At that point he was not interested in discussing spiritual matters, so she just visited him. He did tell her that he considered himself agnostic. He said he believed there might be a God someplace, but he was not sure. He had gone to Sunday school as a boy, but he really did not see how any of those stories applied to him. He was doing all right on his own—a successful lawyer, a nice family, two cars and a boat.

"But now the cancer seems more serious?" Nell ventured. "And scary?"

He nodded. "I feel like I'm at the end of myself. I'm just torn up inside. Everybody is trying to comfort me. My wife is being so patient and good. But she can't really help. A hospital counsellor came up, and I tried to talk with him, but all he asked me was how did I *feel* about all this. How does he think I feel? Just lousy, thank you."

He reached for a cigarette. "The doctor says it doesn't matter now whether I smoke or not." He shrugged, then threw the cigarette back down on the table.

"Nell," he said softly, "I know you're a Christian, and you seem so confident and sure. Is there any hope in the Bible? Any comfort? How can a person be comforted by stories and legends?"

Nell took a deep breath. She prayed silently, *Give me the words, Lord.*

"Douglas," she said. "We know each other pretty well by now. You know I'll be absolutely honest with you. I can't change your circumstances or make your cancer go away. I can encourage you about your chemotherapy, and tell you about people who have done well with it, but I can't change the fact that the cancer has metastasised. I can't comfort you." She looked at him squarely. "But I can introduce you to Someone who can." Nell got out a small Bible.

"There is comfort here, Douglas. Real comfort for the deepest part of your being. This Book is not made up of myths and legends. It is God's Word. He gave it to us so that we could know him. It's not like any other book that was ever written. At least forty authors were used by God to give us this Book. They were from all walks of life—a king, a shepherd, a physician, a tax collector, a fisherman. These people wrote over a period of about sixteen hundred years, yet what they wrote is in one accord. Now tell me, Douglas, do you think you could find forty people anywhere who are in total agreement?"

He laughed. "All I've seen people do is argue," he said.

"All the books of the Bible form one single Book because they are connected by a central theme—Jesus Christ. It's like the string in a strand of pearls. When the string is missing, the pearls are not connected. Many people try to use the Bible without understanding the central theme, and the stories seem as disconnected as the scattered pearls. All the way through this wonderful Book, we are told of God and his plan to bring us to himself. As a matter of fact, Revelation 4:11 says that God has made us for himself. That's why he created us. He loves you, Douglas, and wants more than anything for you to come to him."

Uneasily Douglas looked around the room.

"You see, Douglas," Nell continued, "God created man to have perfect fellowship with him. But when the first man sinned by being disobedient, he broke that beautiful relationship with God, not only for himself but also for all generations to follow. This is why our physical bodies get sick and die, and this is why we are spiritually separated from God. God is holy, and man is sinful. That situation causes a great gulf between God and man."

"But I don't feel like I'm so bad," said Douglas. "I've tried to be honest in my business dealings. I'm good to my family, and I've tried to live by high moral standards. Higher than most people, anyway. I really don't think I'm all that sinful."

Nell looked up Romans 3:23 in her Bible.

"Read this," she said.

" 'For all have sinned, and come short of the glory of God.' "

"Who has sinned?" Nell asked.

"All?"

"All. That verse also mentions one of the ways we've sinned. Can you tell me what it is?"

"Do you mean by coming short of the glory of God? Is that how I've sinned?"

"We've all fallen short of God's perfection, Douglas. Every one of us. From the murderer on death row to your sweet grandmother—all have sinned. The so-called goodness of man at its best can't begin to reach the implicit standard of God's holiness—only Christ qualifies. People are constantly trying to reach God through their own efforts, by going to church, being 'religious', being 'good'. Our efforts are just not enough, Douglas. Hard as we try, we still fall short of the holiness of God."

"Now, wait a minute, Nell. I thought that being a good person was what religion was all about. Isn't that it? If we can't be good enough, no matter how hard we try, then that's pretty depressing."

"It would be," said Nell, "except that God loves us so much that he has a way to satisfy his perfect holiness while providing a way for us to come to him. He became a Man, Jesus the Man, very Man and very God. He was born to die for lost humanity. When Jesus died on the cross, he paid the penalty for all our sins. All that is required of us is that we accept what he already has done."

"That can't be," Douglas said. "It's too simple, too easy. There's surely more to it than that."

"It's simple, Douglas, but it's not always easy. It's simple enough that everyone can understand it. But we tend to complicate it and make it hard. We'd much rather *do* something than accept what God has already done. It appeals to our pride to think we might do something to deserve this great gift. Read Ephesians 2:8, 9."

" 'For by grace are ye saved through faith; and that not of yourselves: it is the gift of God: not of works, lest any man should boast.' "

"You see, Douglas, as we invite him into our hearts as Saviour, we are wrapped in a robe of righteousness, his righteousness, and we're given the authority to be called God's very own children. When we know for sure that we belong to him, that we are his, then we have real hope. It's hope that in no way depends on our circumstances. It doesn't depend on biopsy reports, X-ray results, or anything else. It goes beyond today or tomorrow, and he opens our eyes to spiritual matters so we can have true understanding of his Word. Best of all, we can face death with confidence, knowing that because of him we have life that never ends. Death no longer holds the terror for us that it did before, because we know that we have eternal life, starting the moment we accept Christ.

"We can have real comfort and hope, Douglas, but it has to be God's way. Would you like to receive Jesus right now as your own Saviour and Lord?"

"It sounds good, Nell. It really does. But I want to think about it for a while."

"I can understand that, Douglas. Just remember that God loves you and wants the very best for you. I'll be praying for you."

The small Bible Nell left with Douglas had several verses marked in the front. Although he had seldom used a Bible, he found the book names listed and was able to slowly and methodically look up each verse. As he read, Douglas became more and more excited.

John 3:16 told him that God loved him so much he gave his only Son that whoever would believe in him would not perish but have eternal life.

John 1:12 told him that a person could become a child of God by accepting his Son. Revelation 3:20 told him that Christ was standing at the door of his life, knocking. All he had to do was open the door to his life, and Christ would come in. First John 5:11, 12 told him that God gives us eternal life, and this life is in his Son. The person who has the Son has life; the person who does not have the Son does not have life. Isaiah 61:10 told him that the Lord would cover him with a robe of righteousness.

That's it, he said silently. *That's it! God has already done all this for me. Yes, Jesus, yes! I am a sinner, but you died for me. I accept what you did on Calvary as payment for my sin. Come into my life now and be my Saviour and Lord. Thank you, Lord, thank you.*

On that day, Douglas Evans found the true meaning of *hope.* He knew that whatever else might happen, he could be sure his life would not end with the death of his body. He would be with Christ throughout all eternity, and death would merely be the passageway from this life into something much better.

Douglas found too that he could walk with the Lord on a day-by-day basis. He knew that, even if all his earthly hopes failed him, he could depend upon the blessed Controller of all things.

9

OUR HUMAN EMOTIONS

I waited patiently for the LORD; and he inclined unto me, and heard my cry. He brought me up also out of an horrible pit, out of the miry clay, and set my feet upon a rock, and established my goings. And he hath put a new song in my mouth, even praise unto our God: many shall see it, and fear, and shall trust in the Lord (Psalm 40:1–3).

When cancer is diagnosed, its victims are often flung into a "horrible pit" of despair.

When Nell Collins learned that the mole on her back was a malignant melanoma, she screamed and cried as she drove home from the doctor's office. She screamed hysterically for three days. Like so many other cancer patients, she thought that the diagnosis of cancer meant positively that she was going to die—and soon.

Though it sometimes happens that cancer patients do die soon after diagnosis, it is just as true that hundreds of thousands of cancer patients return to full, productive lives after diagnosis and treatment. Millions of people who had cancer diagnosed and treated at least five years ago are alive and well today. They are considered cured of the disease and lead normal, active lives.

Millions more cancer patients, however, live for years not cured. Instead they fight this disease every moment with repeated surgery, various kinds of treatments, chemotherapy, and a strong will to live. Many more patients are fighting a losing battle with cancer than have been cured.

It takes courage to be a long-term cancer patient. Battling a devious enemy that remains elusive and relatively unknown becomes as much an emotional struggle as a physical one.

NEGATIVE FEELINGS

The cancer patient and those who love him may be discouraged, worried, depressed. There will be days when fear is powerful. The cancer patient may have times when the medication he is taking makes him despondent. He probably will feel tremendous resentment that this terrible thing should happen to him.

All of us experience the full range of human emotions— from sadness to joy, from hate to love, from panic to peace. We recognise that some of these emotions are positive, healthy, good. Others can be negative, defeating, destructive.

Emotions such as depression and sadness are not always wrong. Jesus grieved in Gethsemane. He wept, groaned, and felt rejected. God gave us our emotions. If we could not feel sorrow, could we recognise joy?

Worry and fear are human. They are emotions that are almost a reflex action in some situations. If you are driving a car and suddenly see a lorry heading straight for you, you will most certainly be fearful. When cancer is diagnosed, not to know some fear and anxiety would be unnatural.

Of course, a teenager with a brain tumour will be depressed. He sees his friends healthy and having fun, and he feels cheated out of life. He would not be human if he did not feel some distress.

Every human being will experience negative emotions.

The danger is that these negative emotions can rule us, rob us of our joy, and ruin our sweet fellowship with the Lord.

Even Christians who have walked close to the Lord are subject to these negative emotions. Family members might be surprised to see a normally tranquil Christian react with a burst of rage or deep depression.

Other patients may put on a fantastic performance, attempting to gloss over their real feelings so that the family members will not be upset. This kind of patient is typically (but not necessarily) a mother who is trying to protect her family. Then the family members, too, try to protect the patient from anything unpleasant, so the result is usually a great deal of playacting and virtually no communication. The family members deceive themselves into thinking that the patient is handling it "just fine". If the negative emotions are not faced squarely, they become snarled in a web that is nearly impossible to untangle.

Some Christians have the idea that they can handle these negative emotions by virtue of their great self-control. So they clench their fists, grit their teeth, and mutter through tight lips, "I will not be angry; I will not be afraid." No matter how hard we try, our self-control is no match for these negative emotions. Only God is strong enough, and his Holy Spirit lives within every believer with the power to defeat the negatives. But the believer must be absolutely honest about his inability to fight the negative emotions on his own, and he must allow the Holy Spirit to be in control of his life, emotions and all.

A Christian especially may feel that a negative emotion is wrong and therefore may deny having that emotion. Denial, however, does not rid the person of the negative emotion; denial pushes it "underground".

To face a negative emotion squarely, a person must (1) identify it, (2) acknowledge it, (3) see it as God sees it, (4) when it is sin, confess it as such, and (5) ask God to replace the negative emotion with a positive one by the power of the Holy Spirit.

What are these negative emotions with which the cancer patient may have to contend?

Fear. Every cancer patient experiences a degree of fear. The dictionary calls fear a "painful feeling of impending danger". This emotion wears many disguises: anxiety, doubt, timidity, indecision, superstition, withdrawal, loneliness, overaggression, worry, feelings of inferiority, cowardice, hesitance, depression, haughtiness, shyness.[1]

Sometimes our fear is so great we become afraid of our fear. Eileen Tiedt in *Nursing Forum* describes the process in this manner:

> Individuals respond to fear and anxiety in different ways. They may withdraw, become depressed, become demanding. Fear and a high level of anxiety may be interpreted by the patient to mean he or she is losing emotional control. Loss of self-control is a crucial threat to the integrity of any person; thus, the lack of control, generated by the original fear, increases the fear and a vicious circle ensues.[2]

Perhaps you are afraid of God. If the wrath of God is all you know about him, then you are seeing an incomplete picture of his character. He is both perfect justice and perfect love. Those who refuse to meet his conditions have good reason to fear him, but those who have basked in the wonder of his loving-kindness through his Son know that there is no fear in love.

It really helps to memorise Scripture verses, so that when fear strikes you have this comfort readily available. Elsa, a Christian in fellowship with the Lord, at times could not breathe because of her lung cancer, and she panicked when those times came. Elsa memorised a few verses, and they helped calm her during frightening moments.

"Fear not: for I have redeemed thee, I have called thee by

thy name; thou art mine. When thou passest through the waters, I will be with thee; and through the rivers, they shall not overflow thee: when thou walkest through the fire, thou shalt not be burned; neither shall the flame kindle upon thee. For I am the Lord thy God, the Holy One of Israel, thy Saviour" (Isa. 43:1–3).

"God is our refuge and strength, a very present help in trouble. Therefore will not we fear, though the earth be removed, and though the mountains be carried into the midst of the sea" (Ps. 46:1, 2).

"For God hath not given us the spirit of fear; but of power, and of love, and of a sound mind" (2 Tim. 1:7).

"What time I am afraid, I will trust in thee" (Ps. 56:3).

Anger. "I shook my fist at God and screamed at him!"

Do not be surprised if you find yourself angry because you have cancer. You may find that the object of your anger is God, because he has allowed this illness to come into your life.

Anger is manifested in a number of ways: envy, intolerance, criticism, revenge, hatred, rebellion, jealousy, unforgiveness, bitterness, indignation, wrath, quarrelling.[3] Anger is the forerunner of resentment. When you are angry with God, a wall of resentment builds, affecting not only your fellowship with him but with those around you.

When we are angry with God for allowing cancer in our lives, we are saying, "God, I don't like the way you are running things. You let this miserable thing happen to me, and I don't like it."

Psychologists have found that unresolved anger always plays a part in depression and usually is involved, in some way, in other kinds of mental and emotional illness. Doctors now see a direct link between anger and many physical illnesses. Ulcers, high blood pressure, heart trouble, and numerous other physical ailments have been linked to anger.

In order to resolve anger, a person must first acknowledge that he is angry. Anger that is denied leads in an insidious way to resentment. A person can harbour resentment without being consciously aware that he is doing so. Acknowledging anger and confessing it when it is sin has a remarkable dissipating effect.

Depression. Depression is a common problem in our society. Tranquillisers and antidepressants are sold in huge volumes both legally and illegally—indicating that depression is not a condition limited to the cancer patient. After a few days or weeks, tranquillisers themselves often cause depression.

Watching the evening news is enough to make a person mildly depressed. The world is full of sad, tragic, and miserable circumstances.

Of course, this problem of depression can be caused by a physical abnormality or a chemical or hormonal imbalance. If you are depressed, you should first check with your doctor to see if there is a physical cause. Powerful chemotherapy drugs sometimes cause depression, also.

Most depression, however, is mental or emotional in nature. Usually it is the result of unresolved anger or fear with resentment added.

People, in a very general sense, tend to be either anger-prone or fear-prone. One person will respond with anger to a given set of circumstances, while another person will respond with fear to the same set of circumstances. Fear and anger are powerful emotions and, if repressed, naturally lead to a state of depression.

It is important to try to uncover the underlying cause of the depression. Dr Roy W. Menninger, president of the Menninger Foundation, says, "You can't jolly people out of depression, or shame them out of it. In most people, depression is a kind of repressed anger, and these people have given up any effort to express that anger."[4]

In *How to Win Over Depression*, Tim LaHaye says that sickness itself is one of the major causes of depression.

> Everyone has his breaking point. We have already seen that some people can endure more pressure or depression-producing circumstances than others. But whatever your tolerance for depression, it will be lowered through illness. Protracted periods of illness make you even more vulnerable. . . . In addition, when a person is weakened or debilitated by illness, things that would ordinarily not bother him tend to be unduly magnified. It is probably easier to drift into self-pity during an illness than at any other period.[5]

LaHaye gives this subject thorough treatment in his book, and I recommend it for anyone who finds depression a problem. See also *Defeating Despair and Depression* by Matilda Nordtvedt (Chicago: Moody, 1974).

Severe depression can result in despair. The thought of facing the future with all its uncertainties may seem too much to bear. You, as the patient, may come to the point where you believe your family would be better off without you. You might feel it would be better for everybody if you just jumped out the window.

Suicide causes family members more terrible grief than any other cause of death. The very ones you want to protect from the ordeal of your debilitating illness will suffer much more if you take your own life. You will burden them with a heart-wrenching sense of guilt if you take such action.

If anyone reading this book is experiencing these feelings, I urge you to look to Christ for the answer to your depression. He can give you hope; he can meet your every need. God has something wonderful planned for you. Your situation may seem terrible and hopeless, but God can use it, somehow, in a marvellous way.

Discouragement. Armin Gesswein tells the story of two frogs in *How to Overcome Discouragement*: "Somehow they both fell into a large cream crock. The one frog croaked right away! Down he went. He said, 'I've had it!' The second frog said to himself, 'Well, if I'm going down, I'm not going to go down without a struggle anyhow.' So he kicked and paddled and churned . . . and the first thing he knew he was sitting on a cake of butter! Which frog are you?"[6]

"The Lord God of thy fathers hath said unto thee; fear not, neither be discouraged" (Deut. 1:21).

"Let us lay aside every weight, and the sin which doth so easily beset us [could this be discouragement?], and let us run with patience the race that is set before us, looking unto Jesus, the author and finisher of our faith" (Heb. 12:1, 2).

Doubt. Illness may lead us to question things we had taken for granted before: Does God exist? Does he love me? How would he let this happen? Is Christ the only way to God?

God welcomes honest searching. Christianity is based on historical fact, not on the speculations of men. It will not collapse under close examination. Ask your questions. Seek your answers. Talk to God about your doubts and questions. Ask him for the wisdom that will lead you to him. Search the Bible for answers. Find out for yourself what Scripture says about what you are questioning. Your questions and reliance upon the truth of God's Word may lead you to a new level of commitment. If you are struggling with accepting the evidence supporting the Christian faith, read Josh McDowell's *More Than a Carpenter* (Tyndale, 1977) and Robert A. Laidlaw's *The Reason Why* (Moody, n.d.).

Honest questioning is healthy. But be careful—you can develop the habit of doubting (and consequently not believing), and that habit is hard to break.

You will have questions that cannot be answered, because God has not chosen to tell us everything. Many, many things will remain a mystery in this world—in both the physical realm and the spiritual. "The secret things belong unto the Lord our God: but those things which are revealed belong unto us and to our children for ever" (Deut. 29:29).

God has given us enough information so that the most intellectual person can be satisfied, yet he leaves enough out so that we all must have faith without fully understanding. Many times we would join the anguished father who said to Jesus, "Lord, I believe; help thou mine unbelief" (Mark 9:24).

Worry. Worry eats away at your heart, mind, and spirit. It damages your sense of well-being. Worry is a hand-maiden to cancer: so many things are not known; so many tests have to be run; it takes so long to get the results.

Cancer causes a mother to worry about who will take care of the children while she is ill, or if she should die. Cancer causes anxiety about physical appearance. Mastectomy patients especially worry about how their husbands will react to the fact of their breast surgery.

Every cancer patient hopes he will be cured, but the worry that the cancer will someday return never goes away. Generally, those who work with cancer patients say that a patient is "cured" after five years without symptoms of the disease. This is a simple rule of thumb, however; cancer has been known to recur after that length of time. Unfortunately, every cancer patient has to live out an allotted time to see whether or not he can be called "cured". Worry results.

Cancer care is expensive, and worry about money can plague not only the cancer patient but everyone in the family.

Your worry can destroy you. But the Bible offers an alternative:

Don't worry about anything; instead, pray about everything; tell God your needs and don't forget to thank him for his answers. If you do this you will experience God's peace, which is far more wonderful than the human mind can understand. His peace will keep your thoughts and your hearts quiet and at rest as you trust in Christ Jesus. (Philippians 4:6, 7 TLB)

Regret or remorse. "If only I had gone to the doctor sooner—"

"Why did I say those mean things to him? I should have known he was sick—"

"If only—if only—if only—"

Regret is a wasted emotion. It is futile; in no way can it change things. What is done is done, and no amount of self-recrimination can change the past. Regret and remorse are guilt feelings in disguise. If not resolved, these feelings also lead to depression. See chapter twelve for more information on the difference between *feeling* guilty and *being* guilty.

Of course you have made mistakes. We all make mistakes, and some of those mistakes have heavy consequences. Just remember: you did the very best you could with the information you had at the time.

You can become totally preoccupied with regret. If you have done or said something wrong, confess it to God and *accept his forgiveness.*

Regret seems to be more of a problem for the family members than it is for the cancer patient. A mother may torture herself with real or imagined failings and in the end blame herself for her child's sickness. This is agony beyond belief, and it is not necessary.

As a Christian, you can bring the entire situation before God, commit it to him, and leave it there.

10

LIVING ABOVE CIRCUMSTANCES

The cancer patient sometimes experiences many things that are depressing. Tubes, machines, equipment. Nausea, pain, weakness. Tearstained faces of loved ones. Worry about every ache. Is it the cancer? Hospitals, waiting rooms, treatment centres. Making friends with people, then hearing about their funerals.

Family members, too, are thrust into difficult circumstances. If we look at circumstances, our negative emotions can get a powerful grip on us and take us to the depths of despair.

Christians are not exempt from having the negative emotions discussed in chapter nine. But Christians do have a way of conquering those emotions, a way not available to unbelievers.

THE OLD NATURE

Every person who is born into this world (Christ excepted) has what the Bible calls an "old nature". This old nature is called "the flesh", which is not a reference to our physical bodies. Rather, the flesh is that part of us that is against God. This old nature causes self to be the ruler of the life; it causes sin in the life; it causes active rebellion or indifference toward God. It is also the old nature that causes a person to look to self for solutions to all problems. This elevation of self leads to a philosophy in which the answers to our needs must come from the human realm. If God is recognised at all, he is thought to be far, far away and not much interested in our problems.

The Christian is one who has seen the futility of the self-life. He has recognised that by his own efforts he cannot measure up to God's holy standards, so he has received Christ as his Saviour and Lord. At the moment of this decision, self is dethroned, and Christ becomes the King of the life. God himself, in the person of the Holy Spirit, comes to dwell within, and a permanent, eternal relationship is established. Paul spoke of this permanent relationship when he said, "For I am convinced that neither death, nor life, nor angels, nor principalities, nor things present, nor things to come, nor powers, nor height, nor depth, nor any other created thing, shall be able to separate us from the love of God, which is in Christ Jesus our Lord" (Rom. 8:38, 39, NASB).

THE NEW NATURE

The Christian is given a "new nature", and he is made a new creation. "Therefore if any man be in Christ, he is a new creature: old things are passed away; behold, all things are become new" (2 Cor. 5:17).

The Holy Spirit is possessed by every believer. Often called the Comforter, the indwelling Spirit of God brings glory to Christ and causes our lives to be transformed.

Why is it, then, that so many Christians are living miserable, defeated lives? The problem is that the Christian does not lose his "old nature". As long as he lives in his human body, he has the capacity to sin. It is possible for him to put self back in control of his life. It is to God's glory that he can use weak, failing creatures to accomplish his great works. That is why "we have this treasure in earthen vessels, that the excellency of the power may be of God, and not of us" (2 Cor. 4:7).

The Christian who is not allowing Christ to control his life, to be the very centre of his life, is called in the Bible "carnal," or "fleshly". This means that self is again in control of the life, and the believer is once more wrapped up in himself. This condition may be manifested in many ways—from obvious sin to the tyranny of negative emotions. In any case, self is at the centre of the life. When Paul describes the plight of the carnal Christian in Romans 7, he uses the personal pronouns *I, me,* and *my* more than thirty times. He sums up the miserable state of the carnal Christian by saying, "O wretched man that I am!" (Rom. 7:24).

THE DOUBLE-MINDED MAN

When a believer allows the old nature to be in control, his emotions will definitely be affected. When self is in command of the life, the believer concentrates on his circumstances, and the result is worry, fear, anger, guilt, a critical spirit, resentment, depression, bitterness—any or all of those ugly, negative emotions that are so destructive and can tear us apart.

Many believers live with a constant civil war going on between the old nature and the new nature. James says that this kind of believer is "double-minded" and "unstable in all his ways" (James 1:8). The situation suggests a train with an engine attached to each end. One pulls one way; one pulls the other. As a result, the train is going to be in sad shape.

Any believer who has cancer and does not understand the tremendous struggle between the two natures may find himself shocked at his own emotional response. Larry Gorden is an example of such a case.

"I had been a Christian for several years", he says, "before the diagnosis of lung cancer. I had all kinds of preconceived ideas of how a Christian 'should' be. My life was pretty much on an even keel before the diagnosis. Oh, I had times when my temper would flare, or I'd worry about a business deal. But nothing I couldn't handle, if you know what I mean.

"But when they hit me with that diagnosis, and told me it had already spread to other organs—well, I just went into a tailspin. I was so depressed I couldn't talk or eat or sleep.

"But worse than the depression, I felt so *guilty* about being depressed! I thought Christians were supposed to be joyful, no matter what the circumstances. I had heard about the Christian martyrs who were thrown in the lions' den and sang hymns of praise while the lions were roaring at them. This cancer was a lion roaring at me, all right, but I wasn't singing."

GOD'S PROVISION

Larry did not recognise the power of the old nature to take these negative emotions and make him more or less a slave to them. Because of a visit from Nell Collins, however, he began to recognise that God had made provision for his distress.

"You know, Larry," Nell said, "God understands us far better than we do. And he is so faithful to meet our needs, whatever they are. His Word tells us in 1 John 1:8 that if we say we have no sin, we're deceiving ourselves, and the truth is not in us. That means that it is indeed possible for a Christian to sin. And whether we like the word *sin* or not, we have to know that whatever is not of faith is sin. We are told that in Romans 14:23. So we ask ourselves, What is faith? It is trust, reliance, confidence in God. When we are doubting and fearful and depressed, our emotions are simply pointing to our lack of trust in the God of the universe, who is the blessed Controller of all things."

Nell explained to Larry that God gives us a very simple answer to this problem. We are freed from guilt by claiming the promise of God's Word in 1 John 1:9: "If we confess our sins, he is faithful and just to forgive us our sins, and to cleanse us from all unrighteousness." Confessing means simply to agree with God concerning those negative emotions, see them the way he does. We do not have to *beg* God for forgiveness.

"When Christ died on the cross", Nell said, "every sin of yours and mine was nearly two thousand years in the future. He died for all of our sins, so as Christians we never have to wonder if God will forgive us.

"But as long as we keep making excuses, saying, Well, that's just the way I am, or defending our attitudes, saying, I have a right to feel this way, then our negative emotions will continue to rule us. God wants us to face those emotions squarely, to see them honestly, to recognise them for what they are. Then he wants us to agree with him, saying, Yes, God, I am depressed, and it's because I'm not trusting you. Thank you for your *total forgiveness*."

TRUST IN THE LORD

Nell went on to say that *fear* is often at the root of depression. This fear is sometimes fear of God and what he might do to us. Such a sad concept of the character of God! He wants what is the very best for us. He *loves* us. This kind of fear, again, is evidence of not trusting him.

The Bible says, "Trust in the Lord with all thine heart; and lean not unto thine own understanding" (Prov. 3:5). We may be surprised at our limited understanding of cancer, and how often the doctors have to say, "We just don't know." Many cancer patients are greatly distressed when the doctors do not seem to know which course of treatment would be best.

This is why we have to trust in the Lord with *all* of our hearts. If we lean on our own meagre understanding, we will be miserable indeed.

What does the phrase "trust in the Lord" mean? Christians use these words so much that the expression might sound glib, but what does it really mean? And how can a person go about trusting?

Trust is a simple, childlike quality. Our youngest child loves to go to the swimming pool with her daddy. He stands in the water; and she leaps with a shout of joy off the side of the pool into his waiting arms. This is trust. She knows that he will not fail her. She knows that he is taking care of her.

Suppose she did not have this attitude. Suppose she would cling, crying and wailing, to the side of the pool. Her daddy would not have changed. His strong arms would be waiting there for her, but unless she would *trust* him, he could not comfort her.

If she sees the deep water and lets her mind become filled with thoughts of drowning, if she concentrates on her *fears*, then that sweet, joyful time with her father is lost. She is miserable, and he is saddened by her lack of trust.

Is this not the way it is when we refuse to trust our heavenly Father?

In order for us to really understand how those long-ago Christians could sing with the hot breath of the roaring lions upon them, we must realise that peace in any circumstance comes by placing oneself completely in the hands of the Lord. Sometimes we hang on so desperately to things we consider ours. Our health. Our families. Our future.

The Bible says, "Or do you not know that your body is a temple of the Holy Spirit who is in you, whom you have from God, and that *you are not your own?* For you have been bought with a price: therefore glorify God in your body" (1 Cor. 6:19, 20, NASB, emphasis mine).

We belong to God. We are his. Because we know we can trust him, because we know he is good, because we know he loves us with an everlasting love, then we can give ourselves and all that we love to him. As an act of the will, we relinquish *all* to him.

A LIVING SACRIFICE

Larry Gorden says: "When Nell left that day, I knew exactly what my problem was, and what I must do about it. I knew that my emotions were ruling me, and that I was afraid to trust the Lord with very much of anything. I seemed to remember a verse about offering your body as a living sacrifice, so I looked it up. It was Romans 12:1: 'I beseech you therefore, brethren, by the mercies of God, that ye present your bodies a living sacrifice, holy, acceptable unto God, which is your reasonable service.' I had only heard this verse in connection with becoming a missionary, but God was telling me something very different that day.

"I was literally to give him my body, cancer and all. I was to give him what I thought was my right to be healthy. Then he brought to my mind all the other things I was hanging on to—worry about what the future would hold for my wife and kids, my business, my money, my fear of pain, my worry about being a burden to everyone.

"I took out a sheet of paper and carefully tore it into strips. On each strip, I wrote down one of these things, starting with 'My body'.

"Then, one by one, I presented each of these things to my Lord Jesus. I gave all my worries to him. Then I tore up the papers. I simply could not believe the change this action brought about in my attitude. It was like a load had been lifted from me. All my worries suddenly were *his*, and I was free! My depression was gone, and I couldn't wait until my wife came to visit so I could share this with her.

"Yes, I still have times when I worry or am fearful. But I just say, Lord, why am I worrying about *your* problem? Then I hand it back to him again."

11

FACING DIFFICULT SITUATIONS

Each cancer patient encounters his own difficult situations.
For some, the problem may be purely physical: walking,
eating, talking. For others, the trial might be financial:
inadequate insurance, expensive treatments. For others, the
emotional upheaval is staggering: a paralysing fear of the
future in terms of the cancer itself, an agonising worry
about what will become of the children if death should
occur, deep depression. For some, there are other kinds of
physical difficulties: transportation to and from the doctor's
office for treatments, getting housework done, the inability
to take care of the children's needs, problems connected
with a business interest needing attention that cannot be
given.

Every cancer patient faces some kind of difficult situation
or a combination of several. A number of cancer patients
told me what they considered to be their greatest problems
and what they found to be the most significant help in facing
them. These people are some of the cancer patients Nell
Collins has visited. They are Christians who have known
God's faithfulness in time of trouble.

Remember that each person's cancer is an individual case.
The treatment prescribed for someone else is not necessarily
the right treatment for you. That someone else is getting a
treatment you are not getting does not mean he is getting
too much or that you are getting too little. Perhaps,

however, it will help you to know what others have encountered, and how they have dealt with their problems.

CASE 1

Medical information. Radical mastectomy, left side, followed by an oophorectomy six months later to remove ovaries and eliminate oestrogen. Patient has been having chemotherapy treatment.

Difficult situation. "One of the most trying experiences in this whole ordeal has been having to cope with the fact that the doctors are not always in 100 per cent agreement about every detail. Somehow I thought that surely specialists would have the same opinion regarding treatment. To a nonmedical person it is really frightening when the doctors don't agree with each other.

"In my case, the doctors got into a big discussion about whether or not I should have radiotherapy. It really scared me. All I could do was pray, 'Lord, I don't know what to do—one doctor says I should have radiation, the other doctor says I shouldn't. Help me trust this third doctor with the decision.'

"I asked Dr D. why there was such a difference of opinion between doctors, and he said it is just because there's so much we don't know. I said, 'Well, that's not very comforting to the patients.' He said, 'It's not very comforting to the doctors, either.'"

Comment. In a hospital setting, particularly in a large metropolitan hospital or medical centre, the cancer patient may be seen by several doctors and students. In the technical details of medicine, doctors can and do sometimes have differences of opinion. The patient and family may be greatly upset, as the patient was in this case, by what appears to be a conflict among the doctors regarding proper treatment. Doctors need to realise the importance of this problem and to sort out differences before meeting with the patient.

If a patient or family member hears what seems to be conflicting opinions, he should go to the doctor in charge of the case to clear up any confusion.

CASE 2

Medical information. Dark spot on leg, diagnosed as malignant melanoma. Extensive surgery is required with this type of cancer, because the roots can go very deep.

Difficult situation. "Although I felt well after the surgery, I had a real problem accepting the large, ugly scar on my leg. At least I saw it that way. I thought everyone was staring at it, and I was so embarrassed by it. I wore a covering over it for a year and a half. Finally, Nell told me that I needn't be ashamed of that scar, that I could use it for a testimony.

"It has been amazing to me, since I started going around with the scar showing, the way people have responded. First of all, most people are so wrapped up in themselves that they don't even notice it! But sometimes people ask me about it, and that opens the door for me to be able to share my faith in Christ with them. A few people have even come to know the Lord because we have been able to have these conversations. If I had kept my scar covered, I'd have missed out on these blessings!"

CASE 3

Medical information. Cancer in right breast, which was removed in April 1969. Sixteen cobalt treatments. In

October 1976, left breast removed. Cancer in lymph nodes also. Patient is on chemotherapy.

Difficult situation. "As a double mastectomee, I've had a hard time finding a prosthesis that looks natural and feels comfortable. Some people have the idea that the prosthesis solves all the problems of the mastectomy patient, and this is not true. It is important, I believe, to get up in the morning, get dressed, get my makeup on, and get busy. But without a comfortable prosthesis, I just felt like staying in a dressing-gown all day. It was a real problem for me.

"Now this may not be the solution for everyone, but I began experimenting, trying to make a prosthesis for myself that would feel good and look good. I came up with something that, as far as I'm concerned, is just perfect. I wear a regular bra (though not all brands work out for this); then I make my own form and fit it inside the cup. I make the form from panty hose, cutting a piece eight to ten inches from the top part of the thigh of each leg. Then I tie a knot in the narrow end and trim the excess from the knot. Then I turn it inside out, and the place where the knot is tied becomes the nipple. Then I fill it, using a de luxe filler (available from Beckford Mills in Bradford [phone 0274 651065]). Buy the softest and best quality you can find, and don't use cotton—it won't work. You just work the de luxe filler into the form, the size and shape you need, and wear it inside your bra.

"In my case, making my own forms this way has been such a help. I would have paid almost any price to find a prosthesis that worked for me, and I tried some very expensive ones. I know there are several different kinds of manufactured prostheses, and many women are happy with them. So each woman must do her own experimenting.

"The type of form I make works out best for the double mastectomee. A woman who has lost just one breast has the added problem of balancing not only the size of the breast but also the weight. These forms can be weighted. One woman I know makes a little pouch and fills it with bird seed (believe it or not!), then places the pouch in the form with the de luxe filler. She says it works beautifully! It takes some experimenting, but I've shown many women how to do this, and most of them think it's great!"

CASE 4

Medical information. Cancer of the colon; metastasis to both lungs. Patient is on powerful chemotherapy drugs.

Difficult situation. "My biggest problem is nausea after the chemotherapy injections. As a wife and mother, I feel so guilty because I can't do the things around the house that I normally do. The housework and cooking have been totally taken over by my husband and two daughters. I feel so worthless and like such a drain on them."

Comment. This person is experiencing a situation encountered by many cancer patients. Though the difficult situation is centred in the nausea, three problems actually exist.

The nausea itself. This problem is often a side effect of chemotherapy. It is good to know that the nausea usually does not last more than a few days, and there are drugs to help you get through these days. If the nausea is very severe, call your doctor.

The patient's inability to do work she normally does. This, too, is often the case. The family members simply must help each other through these times or else hire someone to help.

The patient's emotional response. This is the hardest problem. While the first two are difficult, they are unavoidable. The third problem, the negative emotional response to the physical problems, is something that through the power of God can be changed. We can have our eyes on our circumstances and get mired in the misery of it all. We also can, as an act of the will, take our eyes off our circumstances and concentrate on Jesus. Nell Collins shows how Psalm 37 gives a simple plan for trusting in the face of adversity.

Trust (v. 3). First we must trust the Lord for our salvation; then we can trust him daily for everything that comes into our lives.

Delight (v. 4). Christ is at the very centre of the life. All activities, plans, and interests are under his divine control. The deepest joy in life is found in him.

Commit (v. 5). Every thought, every action, every decision is committed to the Lord Jesus. In everything we do, we ask, Will this glorify my Lord?

Rest (v. 7). "The eternal God is thy refuge, and underneath are the everlasting arms" (Deut. 33:27). That is total security, total rest. Even if the whole world explodes in our faces, we can take refuge in him.

Wait (v. 7). Do not try to second-guess. He is in control.

CASE 5

Medical information. Breast cancer. Radical mastectomy on one side, then the other side nine months later. Twenty-five cobalt treatments. After two years, cancer was found by exploratory surgery in liver, gall bladder, intestines, spleen, ovaries. She is having chemotherapy treatment.

Difficult situation. "When I was well, I took the major responsibility for running the home (finances, etc.). At first my husband was frustrated and resented having to take over these areas. He also felt he couldn't work and take care of me at night.

"Another problem is that one son has a profound hearing loss and has limited communication with his father.

"I couldn't drive and had no way to go for my treatment.

"In response to all of these really enormous problems, I almost had an emotional breakdown. I felt all hope was gone. I just went berserk. Through Nell Collins I learned that the Lord is in control of everything, that he loves me, and I can put my trust in him for every detail of my life.

"God has met all of my needs, including providing a friend with an air-conditioned car who takes me for therapy every three weeks. The Lord has brought to me many Christian friends who encourage me and meet my needs at the right time. Some other Christian friends are picking up our son and taking him to a church that has a ministry to the deaf.

"Family members are alternating staying with me at night, and I have a Christian girl staying with me in the daytime. In hours of crisis she offers prayer for me and helps share my burden.

"It is so good to be able to trust the Lord through it all."

CASE 6

Medical information. Cancer is in parotid (salivary) gland. It is being treated by radiotherapy.

Difficult situation. "The most difficult period for me was during the time of the radiotherapy. I had a severe burning-type pain at the back of my mouth. This caused retching and extreme discomfort. Sometimes I wondered if I could bear it.

"It helped me during that time to concentrate on the fact that our earthly trials will not last forever. Because of Jesus Christ I can know that someday, either when I die or when he comes for his church, I'll be with him and suffer no more.

"A verse that gives me great comfort and helps me

concentrate on eternity is Romans 8:18. 'For I reckon that the sufferings of this present time are not worthy to be compared with the glory which shall be revealed in us.' "

CASE 7

Medical information. Breast cancer surgery. Radical mastectomy of the left side.

Difficult situation. "I was only thirty at the time of surgery, and I was concerned about how my husband, Bill, would respond to me. For a long time I felt inadequate to meet his needs sexually. I was so afraid that he was just staying with me out of pity. I thought I was repulsive to him. We were not communicating in any meaningful way.

"Then something wonderful happened. My aunt called and told me, 'Bill called me the day after your surgery and told me that all of this has made him realise how very much he loves you, and how precious you are to him. I don't know if he's been able to share that with you, but I thought you'd like to know.'

"When Bill came home that night, I told him about the conversation with my aunt. We both cried and cried. Then we decided we'd better start communicating, so I just asked him some very direct questions.

"I asked him if seeing the scar was upsetting to him and if he would prefer I keep it covered during times of making love. He said that he didn't mind seeing the scar, that his love for me wasn't based on whether I had breasts or not. You'll never know how much it meant to me to have him express that in words.

"For my own sake, I went out and bought several pretty nighties. I found that I was more at ease if the scar was covered, even if it didn't matter to Bill. I took time to choose ones that would be especially attractive, and ones that I could camouflage with a form pinned in the front. You can't believe what a boost it was to my morale. All of that may seem to some to be very unimportant, but it really helped me feel better about myself."

CASE 8

Medical information. Suffering is nothing new to this cancer patient. Before her cancer was diagnosed, she had been hospitalised forty-seven times. A severe fall had caused permanent nerve damage in her back, and she has suffered chronic pain for seventeen years.

Difficult situation. Chronic pain, though in this case not connected with cancer, is extremely difficult to handle. She describes her pain on a scale range of one to ten, one being very mild discomfort and ten being acute.

"Fighting pain," she says, "is a daily battle. When I'm fighting pain, I tend to dread it for tomorrow, for next week, for next month, and next year. It seems so hopeless and is made worse by my secret resentments.

"There are plenty of 'Job's miserable comforters' to make my problem more complex. There are also those who, out of love for me, think they have to sympathetically agree with me no matter what I say or how I act. This is not good for me either.

"A study of early church history showed me that there were many who suffered far more than I was suffering, and they willingly chose to do so for Christ. It was, indeed, their 'cross'. I did not choose my suffering for the cause of Christ. But I can be victorious and magnify Christ in my pain. He can use me and my pain to glorify himself. And this has been my daily prayer.

"To apply these truths to where I am now, living in a real

world, with real people, and feeling real pain, I have come to some practical conclusions. They work for me.

1. Start the day with God (prayer; Bible reading).
2. Define my physical capabilities for that day.
3. Set realistic but God-honouring goals. This I do on paper in order of priority.
4. Make an honest attempt to meet these goals, even if I don't feel like it.
5. Be involved with people when at all possible. Serve *their* needs.

"The above suggestions make it possible for me to cope with pain in the scale range of up to five or six. When pain is in the eight to ten range, that is something else again. Many of my hospitalisations have been because of pain of the most severe nature. But it is still possible to be triumphant. A quiet confidence does help the pain to be more treatable. I know it works for the believer who is looking to Christ on a moment-by-moment basis. I know it works because, through the power of God, I have never lost my temper with a clumsy nurse or aide. Yet I have heard the unbeliever in pain curse God and all those who come near him.

"The more that happens to this body of mine, the more I'm convinced of his very great love for me. I've been in crisis before, and I *know* his grace is sufficient."

CASE 9

Medical information. "In 1973 I had a mastectomy and three months later, an oophorectomy (removal of ovaries). I did have positive lymph nodes diagnosed at that time. Before cobalt treatments, bone and liver scans were run (both negative). I had cobalt for a month, then checkups every six months for the next three years. Then I began having a very stiff neck and back stiffness and pain. A bone scan showed cancer had started from head to pelvis all down the right side. They decided to try male hormone pills. After two months another bone scan showed the cancer had spread all down the left side. I was switched to chemotherapy injections. I was in bed for many weeks with back pain, stiffness, soreness. I could do no housework. After a blood transfusion when my red count got too low, I suddenly felt fine. No pain. I started doing a few things, and I spent part of each day out of bed. The next bone scan showed slight improvement, and no massive spreading."

Difficult situation. "The hardest thing to adjust to was being confined to bed, unable to do anything. I felt very depressed and sorry for myself. My four daughters really pitched in and took over cooking, cleaning, washing, and so forth. This wasn't easy for them with their school schedules.

"I realised the Lord had given me a lot of time to myself, and I made use of it by reading the Bible. I listened to Christian radio and tapes friends brought me. Our church family meant so much to me—their cards showing their love and concern, visits from the pastor, food brought over to help out. I enjoyed reading Christian books of how others faced problems. Through reading *Joni* (Send the Light Trust 1983), the story of a young girl who became a quadriplegic after a diving accident, I realised how unlimited I really was while in bed. She said she couldn't cry because there was no one to blow her nose. I had no such problem. Tears flowed, but I realised that God gives us the strength to bear whatever problems we have.

"I was not a Christian at the time of the original mastectomy, though I thought I was. A real depression showed me I was missing something in life, and I searched for it. I visited a Bible-believing church and heard, 'With Christ you have no past, you have only a future.' This was what I needed to hear. I attended church regularly, listened,

learned, and then I accepted Christ as my Lord and Saviour.
Life has been so different since then. I can depend on Christ
for help at all times, whether for relief from pain or help
when I just don't want to go and get a chemotherapy
injection! At times I still struggle, trying to handle things
myself instead of turning myself completely over to him.
He's teaching me he is far better at handling situations than I
am.

"I have been a Christian two years now, and I realise how
withdrawn and self-pitying I probably would have become,
trying to handle cancer on my own.

"It's hard, knowing I'll probably never be free of the
cancer, but with Christ's help I face each day knowing he is
in control of everything."

A LETTER OF COMMITMENT

A difficult situation often mushrooms in enormity because
it is compounded by our emotional response to that
situation. No matter what the physical circumstances might
be, the emotional trauma can be lessened by committing
those circumstances to the care of the sovereign Lord. Nell
Collins sometimes suggests writing a letter of recommit-
ment to God, a letter that is based on the assurance that he is
doing in our lives that which is for our good and his glory.
Though the circumstances may not change, this kind of
commitment can change a person's attitude toward difficult
situations.

The following is Nell's own personal letter to God. If it
expresses the needs of your heart, you may adopt it as your
own.

Dear God,
   Because I know you through faith in the Lord Jesus Christ,
your Word tells me that I belong to you as your child.

I believe, according to your Word, that you will do everything in my life for my eternal good and for your glory.

And so, because I trust you to be perfect in your dealings with me, I make total surrender of my life to you.

I give you every personal desire that I have for my life. If you choose to give me the privileges of long life and good health, then I will use those gifts to honour your name. I will not ask for those privileges unless you would see fit to give them to me for your glory.

If you deem it wise to give me that which *seems* less than perfect to me, in my humanness, then it is my intent to trust you for those things that I cannot understand. I will thank you for working out your plan for my life so that I will be conformed to the image of the precious Lord Jesus Christ. I will depend upon you to give me grace to always glorify you in the midst of *whatever* you choose for me.

It is my intent not to resent anything you allow to come into my life, even when I can't see what you are doing with me, nor can I understand what you are intending for my tomorrows.

Along with the apostle Paul, I would express before you my desire that Christ be magnified in my body, whether by life or by death.

Lord Jesus, I need you to keep me true to this commitment and to show me immediately when I deviate from it.

Because of your perfect trustworthiness, I trust you completely.

In Jesus's name. Amen.

Signed _____

Date _____

12

WHY ME, GOD?

The young mother, Denise, looks drawn and pale. Sleepless nights spent in the lounge at the hospital have given her an all-consuming weariness. Her baby, approaching his second birthday, has been fighting cancer most of his life. After the baby underwent difficult weeks of radiotherapy and chemotherapy, the cancer was found to have spread; surgery revealed dozens of new, inoperable tumours. In a medical sense, the outlook is not good.

Denise is cried out, worn out, prayed out.

She is a Christian; she has experienced the joy of knowing Christ and following him. She turned to Christ when her son became ill; she prayed fervently for his recovery. And now, unless an outright miracle happens, her son is going to die.

"I think maybe I could bear it," she says softly, "if I only knew *why* this had to happen. Why does my innocent little baby have to die? Why can't he have a chance to grow up and live a full life? And why does this have to happen to me? Is God punishing me for some horrible sin in my life?" She reviews her life, remembering past sins. Has God not forgiven her? Does he not love her? Why is he allowing this to happen? Why? Why?

THE INEVITABLE QUESTION

The anguish of cancer always leads to the inevitable question, Why me, God?

The question seems to be nearly a reflex; even people who do not know God or who doubt his existence ask it. When tragedy strikes, no matter what kind of "philosophy" or "religion" we have, that inborn God-consciousness is awakened. Even without biblical knowledge or theological concepts, we sense that he has allowed this tragedy and that he has a reason for it.

I believe that our physical sufferings are sometimes a consequence of the way we live. Scientists have shown a direct link between smoking and lung cancer, so if a person smokes, he risks lung cancer as a consequence. In the same way, an alcoholic risks cirrhosis of the liver. Certain chemicals are known to cause cancer, so if a person lives or works with those chemicals, cancer may result.

We reap what we sow, and evidence keeps mounting that we have sown an environment fraught with cancer-producing elements. Everything from saccharin to chemically treated pyjamas for children has been suggested as a cancer cause. One of the side effects of modern technology appears to be an increase in cancer-causing agents. They are part of our world.

On a general level, we can accept the imperfect world in which we live. But on a personal level, in the midst of our own immediate trials and tragedies, the answer to why is not so easy.

WE MAY NEVER KNOW

We may never know in this world why God has allowed a specific problem to come to us. He may not reveal to us exactly how he plans to use this problem. Because of this, we must trust him.

"For My thoughts are not your thoughts,
Neither are your ways My ways," declares the Lord.

"For as the heavens are higher than the earth,
So are My ways higher than your ways,
And My thoughts than your thoughts."
(Isaiah 55:8, 9, NASB)

GOD'S REVEALED PURPOSES

God does, however, let us know some of his purposes in allowing us to suffer. Scripture is quite specific in outlining some of these reasons, and in this chapter we will attempt to look at a few of the Bible's explanations.

In general, we can divide the reasons for our earthly trials into five main groups: (1) to draw unbelievers to God, (2) to correct us—for our eternal profit, (3) to prevent sin, (4) to bring glory to God, and (5) to develop us.

To draw unbelievers to God. People who have never prayed in their lives or have never even thought very much about God may turn to him in time of catastrophe. This, I believe, is one of the reasons God allows us to experience problems, trials, and sickness. During these times we realise how limited our humanity is, and we are drawn to him. I personally believe most of us would not realise our need for him if we never experienced problems. Our natural, human desire for self-sufficiency would keep us from knowing him, and we would be eternally lost.

Maurice Wagner describes this time of reaching out in his book *The Sensation of Being Somebody:* "At these times of unusual stress we become conscious of how strong or how weak our inner security really is. We seem to get in touch with our inner selves best in times of crisis. It is then that we begin to reach for some resource to hold onto, some relationship that is available and reliable."[1]

God uses suffering in the life of an unbeliever to draw that person to himself. It may be hard to see at the time, but he does this in the purest love, for our own *eternal* good.

> I have loved you with an everlasting love;
> Therefore I have drawn you with lovingkindness.
> (Jeremiah 31:3, NASB)

To correct us—for our eternal profit. Believers, too, experience tragedy. "He causes His sun to rise on the evil and the good, and sends rain on the righteous and the unrighteous" (Matt. 5:45, NASB).

The believer seems to have two primary questions when he faces cancer: (1) Do I have this disease because I have sinned? and (2) Does God send disease to punish?

Because these questions so often remain unanswered, many cancer patients are frustrated and guilt-ridden.

First of all, disease is one of the general results of sin on a cursed earth. Your disease is not necessarily the result of your personal sin, but it is the consequence of the sin that entered the world when man first disobeyed God. Disease is a part of life on this planet, and few people live without encountering it. It is not God's fault that we have disease, but he does use disease to further his purposes.

All sin in the life of the believer was paid for upon Calvary's cross nearly two thousand years ago. The just demands of a holy God have been met.

God will not punish a believer for sin that has already been paid for. Christ paid the penalty, and his cry from the cross declared, "It is finished." Christ's death made it possible for sin to be forgiven and removed, as God says, "as far as the east is from the west" (Ps. 103:12). Jesus Christ suffered and died for our sins in our place. God will not punish a second time for those sins.

There is a world of difference between *punishment* and *discipline*. God disciplines and corrects his children as a loving Father, but this discipline is not the same thing as punishment. Punishment looks to the sin; discipline looks to the future of the sinner who has been saved from the penalty of sin by the grace of God. Punishment satisfies the Law; discipline is given in love. Notice the similarities between the words *discipline* and *disciple*. Being a disciple of Jesus Christ requires discipline.

Sometimes Christians stray away from God, disobey him, or ignore him. We often live as though we did not even have a Saviour. When these things happen, we do not lose our relationship with God, but we do lose our fellowship with him.

The Lord may use illness or other seeming tragedy to draw us back into close fellowship with himself. Does this seem cruel?

God is a loving Father. He wants the very best for us. He knows we cannot know the joy of the promised abundant life if we are not in close fellowship with him.

I am reminded of this concept when I see my oldest daughter's long dark hair. Usually she keeps it clean, shining, and combed. Sometimes, though, she lets it go, and then I have to intervene. It is oily and full of tangles and snarls. When she allows me to shampoo it, the cleansing helps greatly. But we have to spend a good deal of time combing out those tangles.

She does not like the combing-out process one bit. She cries, and I know it hurts. I am sorry it hurts, but combing has to be done or the problem will get worse. Sometimes, when it is really bad, she instinctively pulls away from me, causing even more distress. I keep telling her that the combing will hurt less if she will just draw closer to me.

When God has to remove tangles from our lives, do we not often respond the same way? Instinctively, we pull away from him. "Draw near to God and He will draw near to you" (James 4:8, NASB).

Because God sometimes does allow illness to draw a believer back into close fellowship, some people assume that if a person is sick, it must be because of personal sin. Many people have a warped concept of God and see him as a cruel tyrant, eager to strike down anyone who steps out of line. They react to a diagnosis of cancer with, What did I do to deserve this?

Medical science has recognised the tremendous problem of guilt, especially as seen in seriously ill patients. Counsellors spend much time trying to reassure people that there is nothing to feel guilty about, but this approach is often not very helpful. The trend today is to see guilt as the result of an overly severe conscience, or superego. It is true that some people are overly introspective. It is true that some people do feel guilty about circumstances beyond their control.

There are two kinds of guilt. *Feeling* guilty is not *being* guilty. People who want to please God often torture themselves with excessive self-examination. The result of this kind of morbid introspection is total concentration on *self* rather than on Christ, the very One who has freed us from this kind of bondage.

Hannah Whitall Smith in *The God of All Comfort* has described the problem in this manner:

> And yet it has been so constantly impressed upon us that it is our duty to examine ourselves, that the eyes of most of us are continually turned inward, and our gaze is fixed on our own interior states and feelings to such an extent that self, and not Christ, has come at last to fill the whole horizon.
>
> By *self* I mean here all that centres around this great big "me" of ours. Its vocabulary rings out the changes on "I," "me," "my". It is a vocabulary with which we are all very familiar. The questions we ask ourselves in our times of self-examination are proof of this. Am I earnest enough? Have I repented enough? Have I the right sort of feelings? Do I realise religious truth as I ought? Are my prayers fervent enough? Is my interest in religious things as great as it ought to be? Do I love God with enough fervour? Is the Bible as much of a delight to me as it is to others? All these and a hundred more questions about ourselves and our experiences fill up all our thoughts, and sometimes our

little self-examination books as well; and day and night we ring the changes on the personal pronoun "I," "me," "my," to the utter exclusion of any thought concerning Christ, or any word concerning "He," "His," or "Him".[2]

This excessive scrutiny of self is not what God wants for us. If we constantly dwell on self, we will always feel guilty. None of us ever can measure up to the absolute righteousness of God, and the more we look inward the more guilty we will feel. Christ died so that we could be clothed in his righteousness, and we are to look to him.

Other times a person *feels* guilty about things over which he has no control. "Surely, somehow, I could have recognised the symptoms earlier." "Surely, somehow, I could have prevented this disease."

Feeling guilty over an unattainable "somehow" is not what God intends for his children either. A person plagued by this kind of guilt should remember that he did the best he could do with the information he had at the time. He is not omniscient; he could not have seen into the future. Perhaps as he looks back, he sees that things could have been handled better. That is no doubt true. It is always easy to see mistakes in the past. Feeling guilty now, however, does not change things. Accept the reality of the *right now*, and put the past behind you.

Being guilty is another story. Many times we feel guilty because we are guilty. We need first to identify what it is about which we feel guilty.

James Dobson, Ph.D, Associate Clinical Professor of Paediatrics at the University of Southern California, says, "The best way to handle guilt is to face it squarely, using it as a source of motivation for change, where warranted." He suggests that a person troubled by guilt should write down his shortcomings—make a list. "Each item should then be assessed as follows: Is my guilt valid? If so, how? If not, isn't it appropriate that I lay the matter to rest?"[3]

If you find that you are feeling guilty because of real

guilt, you should turn to God in repentance and claim his provision of confession of sin. He has promised to forgive our sins and cleanse us from all unrighteousness.

Psychologist Henry R. Brandt, Ph.D, in *The Struggle for Peace* says:

> Christians, even though they have believed in and received Christ for salvation, still sin. Many Christians hold hatred, fear, resentment, jealousy, malice toward others. As a result, fellowship with those persons and the Lord is broken, joy is lost, God's peace is not enjoyed. Confession of sin and forsaking of one's sinful ways in obedience to the Lord and His Word are necessary if the Christian is to enjoy God's peace.[4]

This is God's answer to the problem of guilt. If we recognise the sin in our lives as sin, confess it to God, and accept his forgiveness, then we should have *no guilt feelings*.

God does sometimes use what seems to be tragedy to bring us back into close fellowship with himself. This is true. But he has many other reasons for allowing trials and hardships in the life of a believer.

To prevent sin. Many, many followers of the Lord walk in close fellowship with him and harbour no unconfessed sin. These Christians, too, experience trouble and heartache. They can be sure that God has some other purpose in allowing them to suffer.

God sometimes uses weakness, infirmity, or disease as a preventive measure. Paul had his "thorn in the flesh," which God allowed in order to keep him humble ("lest I should be exalted above measure," 2 Cor. 12:7). Our pride, even spiritual pride, can cause us to get out of fellowship with God. To prevent that, God will sometimes allow us to have problems that seem to have no solution. These remind us of our inadequacy, of our dependence upon him.

To bring glory to God. Physical problems are also used by God to bring glory to himself. According to John 9, when Jesus encountered a blind man, the disciples assumed that the cause of the man's blindness was personal sin: "Master, who did sin, this man, or his parents, that he was born blind? Jesus answered, Neither hath this man sinned, nor his parents; but that the works of God should be made manifest in him" (John 9:2, 3).

Jesus then brought sight to sightless eyes. The man was born blind that he might bring glory to God and help all people understand that Jesus of Nazareth was more than mere man.

Job lost everything—his family, his wealth, his health. God wanted to show Satan that his people did not need to have happy circumstances in order to trust him. At first Job moaned, groaned, and chafed (responding very humanly), but in the midst of his trials he showed his faithfulness and ultimate trust in God by saying, "And as for me, I know that my Redeemer lives" (Job 19:25, NASB).

Your battle with cancer might be a way of bringing tremendous glory to God. Have you ever considered that possibility? God may be using your faith right now to bring others to himself. Such an exciting way for the Lord to bring glory to himself!

> And He put a new song in my mouth,
> a song of praise to our God;
> Many will see . . .
> And will trust in the Lord.
>
> (Psalm 40:3, NASB)

To develop us. Yet another reason for illness in the life of the Christian is the one mentioned most often in Scripture: the development of the believer. This idea is brought out so many times and in so many ways that we probably could never examine them all. We may take just a brief look at some of the ways in which God can use physical problems to develop his child.

To bear fruit. Sometimes we must suffer so that we can bear fruit.

> Break up your fallow ground
> And do not sow among thorns.
>
> (Jeremiah 4:3, NASB)

Have you ever tended a garden? It takes a tremendous amount of digging and ploughing of the hard, unyielding soil. The gardener must spend time working with that soil if it is ever to bring forth fruit. If it could, the soil might complain that the gardener is being too rough. Also weeds must be removed if fruit is going to be produced. Sometimes the plant needs pruning. If just left alone, the ground would stay hard and unproductive, the weeds and insects would take over, and there would be no fruit.

God is our Gardener. He lovingly harrows the soil in our lives, weeds out the old unproductive ways, prunes back the branches of bitterness and strife. He wants us to be productive. We can have neither the fruit of the Spirit—love, joy, peace, patience, kindness, goodness, faithfulness, gentleness, self-control (Gal. 5:22, 23, NASB)—nor the fruit of new souls won to the Lord if we do not allow God to be the Gardener of our hearts.

To produce growth. Our suffering is used by God to produce spiritual growth. "All discipline for the moment seems not to be joyful, but sorrowful; yet to those who have been trained by it, afterwards it yields the peaceful fruit of righteousness" (Heb. 12:11, NASB).

To help others see faith during trials. Hebrews 11 gives us a look into the way God sees faith. Many heroes of the faith—Abel, Enoch, Noah, Abraham, Isaac, Jacob, Joseph, Moses, Joshua, Rahab, and others—are commended because they *believed God.* We are encouraged by the faith they showed during their earthly trials. Others are encouraged by our faith.

To produce patience. "We glory in tribulations also: knowing that tribulation worketh patience" (Rom. 5:3).

To make us more Christlike. "For whom He foreknew, He also predestined to become conformed to the image of His Son, that He might be the first-born among many brethren" (Rom. 8:29, NASB).

To make us sympathetic. "The God of all comfort; who comforteth us in all our tribulation, that we may be able to comfort them which are in any trouble, by the comfort wherewith we ourselves are comforted of God" (2 Cor. 1:3, 4).

To learn submission. Sometimes we suffer to help us learn that we must give ourselves completely to God so that he might work out his purposes through us. The Lord told Jeremiah to go down to the potter's house so that Jeremiah could hear what he had to say: "O house of Israel, cannot I do with you as this potter? saith the Lord. Behold, as the clay is in the potter's hand, so are ye in mine hand" (Jer. 18:6).

A young mother I shall call Jennifer worked through her own personal question, Why me, God? She was stricken with cancer of her vocal cords that progressively involved her tongue and oral cavity. She had radical surgery that was disfiguring. She had to have her tongue removed, which meant she could not talk to her husband, Joe, or her two little girls. She could not even write a note to her youngest child, a little girl of four who had not yet learned to read.

Shortly before she died, Jennifer helped her pastor prepare her funeral message, part of which was a letter she had written to her husband:

There are those who see in the hard things of life the discipline of a loving Father. God's supreme punishment is when God lets us alone as unteachable, incurable, and blind. The Christian knows that whatever comes to him or her comes from a God who is a Father, and that "A father's hand will never cause his child a needless tear." He knows that everything that comes means something, is meant for some purpose, is designed to make him a wiser and better person. We shall cease from self-pity, from resentment, and from rebellious complaint, if we remember that there is no discipline of God that does not take its source in love, and that is not aimed at good.

[Jennifer] learned this. She expressed herself this way in a letter to [Joe] prior to her radical surgery in August. "If this cancer (which I fear and hate) is what is necessary to get my attention and make me turn my life over to God, then it's OK. I should and do praise God for this disaster. As you said, I'm lucky to realise so young what is important in life. This pain and suffering is so short. God has better things planned for me in eternity. I'm grateful that I realise the significance of an afterlife. Praise God that I can be used. I love God and his plan for me."

We may not know in this life exactly why God allows us to suffer. We may know all these reasons, but we may not know which ones apply to our own situation. We must accept this fact. To go on and on, agonising over our question why, is actually not trusting in God's sovereignty.

Our attitude should be this: OK, God, if you want to tell me why this is happening, great. I'd love to know. But, if you choose not to reveal it to me, then that's OK, too. In any case, *I trust you.*

Nell says that because of Christ she can know at least a part of God's purpose. She can glimpse a portion of his great design. She says, "My purpose in living—to know Christ and to make him known. My purpose in suffering—to show Christ strong. My purpose in dying—to be ushered into his very presence and to stay there forever."

So be truly glad! There is wonderful joy ahead, even though the going is rough for a while down here.

These trials are only to test your faith, to see whether or not it is strong and pure. It is being tested as fire tests gold and purifies it—and your faith is far more precious to God than mere gold; so if your faith remains strong after being tried in the test tube of fiery trials, it will bring you much praise and glory and honour on the day of his return. (1 Peter 1:6, 7, TLB)

13

LORD, TEACH US TO PRAY

Sociologists tell us that one of the serious problems of our society is that we do not communicate with one another. We talk *at* each other, but we do not listen; we do not share.

We not only have problems communicating with others; we also have trouble communicating with God. We sometimes talk *at* him, too. We recite memorised lines, or we speak flowery phrases. We would like to be able to talk with God about our deepest fears and doubts, but somehow we are afraid he will not like what we say. So, too often, our prayers become meaningless. Because public prayers are sometimes more like speeches prepared for the audience than for God, many people never hear real prayer.

Real prayer is communicating with the God of the universe. What a privilege! God wants us to be in *constant* communication with him—not just before meals, in church, and during emergencies. Communication is two-way. God speaks to us through his Word as we tell him our deepest heartfelt needs. Prayer is a dialogue between a loving Father and his child.

Andrew Murray says:

> Prayer and the Word of God are inseparable, and should always go together in the quiet time of the inner chamber. *In His Word God speaks to me: in prayer I speak to God.* If there is to be true communication, God and I must both take part. If I simply pray, without using God's Word, I am apt to use my own words and

thoughts. This really gives prayer its power, that I take God's thoughts from His Word, and present them before Him. Then I am enabled to pray according to God's Word. How indispensable God's Word is for all true prayer.[1]

CONDITIONS FOR PRAYER

God gives us four primary conditions for effective prayer:

1. You must be a Christian.
2. You must have no unconfessed sin.
3. You must have a forgiving spirit.
4. You must have faith—belief in the power of God to answer prayer.

It is not surprising that we do not know how to pray or how to make prayer an essential part of our lives. Even the apostles were confused about it.

"One of his disciples said unto him, Lord, teach us to pray" (Luke 11:1). We all need instruction in effective prayer. We need to be taught not only *how* to pray, but to *pray*.

Must be Christian. Jesus answered that disciple with probably the best-known and best-loved prayer of all time, which has come to be known as "The Lord's Prayer".

This prayer begins with reference to the first condition for effective prayer: "Our Father". Only those people who belong to Christ can rightfully call God "Father".

"But as many as received him [Christ], to them gave he power to become the sons of God, even to them that believe on his name: which were born, not of blood, nor of the will of the flesh, nor of the will of man, but of God" (John 1:12, 13).

The first condition of effective prayer, then, is that one be a Christian, a true child of God.

We are also admonished to pray in the name of Christ.

"And whatever you ask in My name, that will I do, that the Father may be glorified in the Son. If you ask Me anything in My name, I will do it" (John 14:13, 14, NASB).

The fullness of the Godhead, the entire Trinity, is involved in our prayers. Our prayers are directed to the Father, in the name of the Son, through the Holy Spirit.

God knows that we are people of the twentieth century. He knows the way we talk to others in natural, everyday language. We should be reverent, of course, but it is unnecessary, I think, to try to pray in seventeenth-century English. We should be as open and honest with God as we are with our best friends. Even more so. We may say *I* in prayer. We may refer to God as *you* instead of *thee* or *thou*. We do not have to be kneeling to pray. We can pray while driving the car or washing the dishes.

Confession. Every time we pray, we should remind ourselves of the fact that sin short-circuits prayer:

> If I regard wickedness in my heart,
> The Lord will not hear.
>
> (Psalm 66:18, NASB)

If we are aware of any sin, no matter how insignificant it seems to us, we should confess that wrong to God. Agree with him concerning it. You do not need to beg his forgiveness—that forgiveness has already been purchased by the blood of Christ. If you are a Christian, God has already made available forgiveness for every sin you ever commit, past, present, and future.

But sin in the life of a believer acts as a barrier between the believer and God. Though our relationship with God can never be broken, our fellowship with him can be disturbed.

One cancer patient said to me, "I know I'm a Christian. But somehow I feel so far away from God."

If you too feel far away from God, it may be that something is wrong in your life—some area is unyielded.

Ask God to reveal to you the barrier that is between you and him. He is faithful, and he will make you aware of the problem. Then you are responsible to confess it to God—agree with him, accept his forgiveness and cleansing—then put it behind you.

Ann Walls, gifted Bible teacher and conference speaker, tells the story of how the well-known verse 1 John 1:9 became real to her. This verse says: "If we confess our sins, he is faithful and just to forgive us our sins, and to cleanse us from all unrighteousness."

Ann tells the story of how, one Sunday morning, she dressed her son for church: clean clothes, shining face, brushed hair. He wanted to go out and play since it was early, so she said, "Sure you can—just don't get dirty."

A few minutes later he came back into the house, covered from head to toe with mud. He looked up at her with big, sad eyes and said, "Oh, Mum, I'm really sorry. You told me not to get dirty, and I did."

Her heart melted, of course, and she said, "OK, son. I forgive you. Now let's go upstairs and get in the bathtub."

Well, did he stiffen! He did not want to get in that bathtub. His problem is often our problem: he wanted *forgiveness*, but he did not want the *cleansing*.

God wants to forgive us and to remove those muddy stains of sin from our lives.

A forgiving spirit. We also must have a forgiving spirit. If someone has wronged us, we will not be able to pray effectively until we have forgiven that person.

"And whenever you stand praying, forgive, if you have anything against anyone; so that your Father also who is in heaven may forgive you your transgressions" (Mark 11:25, NASB).

Faith in God. Finally, to pray effectively we must come to God in faith, believing that he has the *power* to answer our prayers. "And everything you ask in prayer, believing, you shall receive" (Matt. 21:22, NASB).

God does answer believing prayer, provided those things we pray for are in accordance with his will for our lives. The ultimate answers to prayer are under the control of his sovereignty, not our desire.

WHY PRAY?

My son once asked me, "If God already knows everything, why do we pray? He already knows what we want and need."

It is true that an omniscient God, One who knows everything, already knows our problems and needs. We cannot tell him anything he does not already know.

Still, prayer is the provision he has given us. He has *commanded* us to pray. "Pray without ceasing" (1 Thess. 5:17).

He *delights* in our fellowship. "But the prayer of the upright is His delight" (Prov. 15:8, NASB).

Our prayers *glorify* God. "And whatever you ask in My name, that will I do, that the Father may be glorified in the Son" (John 14:13, NASB).

Prayer brings *results*. "Elijah was a man with a nature like ours, and he prayed earnestly that it might not rain; and it did not rain on the earth for three years and six months. And he prayed again, and the sky poured rain, and the earth produced its fruit" (James 5:17, 18, NASB).

When we pray, we follow Christ's *example*. "And in the early morning, while it was still dark, He [Christ] arose and went out and departed to a lonely place, and was praying there" (Mark 1:35, NASB).

Prayer gives us a *peaceful* heart and an *unworried* mind. "Don't worry about anything; instead, pray about everything; tell God your needs and don't forget to thank him for his answers. If you do this you will experience God's peace, which is far more wonderful than the human mind can understand. His peace will keep your thoughts and your hearts quiet and at rest as you trust in Christ Jesus" (Phil. 4:6, 7, TLB).

WHAT DOES PRAYER DO?

Prayer brings God into focus in our lives. Prayer shows our dependence upon him and trust in him. It also makes clear the thoughts and desires of our hearts. It helps us identify and confess areas of sinfulness. Prayer helps us trust God to work out the concerns of our lives in accordance with his will.

Our prayer life will be more effective if we systematically include certain specific elements: praise, confession, thanksgiving, and requests for others and ourselves.

GIVE THANKS IN EVERYTHING?

First Thessalonians 5:18 tells us that we should pray with a thankful heart. "In everything give thanks; for this is God's will for you in Christ Jesus" (NASB).

Give thanks in *everything*? Even now, in the midst of this cancer?

You may not actually *feel* thankful right now, but that is all right. It may take a while for your feelings to catch up with your actions. You can say, God, I don't feel very thankful right now, but I thank you anyway, because I know I can trust you in all circumstances.

It is always difficult to thank God for what seems to be a disaster. To thank God for an approaching death, either one's own death or that of a member of the family, is not an easy thing to do. When it is the death of a child, it is particularly difficult. Yet, once this thanksgiving has been verbalised to God, a peace that passes all understanding does come into the heart of the one who has said, Thank you, Lord.

UNANSWERED PRAYER

Often Christians are frustrated because it seems their prayers are so often not answered. Why is this?

The Bible gives several reasons why prayers seemingly are not answered. Sometimes the Lord says yes, sometimes no, and sometimes wait.

If we ask out of God's eternal purpose, he will have to say no. If we ask something that is not best in terms of our *eternal* good, he will say no.

Our prayer life is most effective when we are controlled by the Holy Spirit, with Christ at the very centre of our lives. God's purposes are higher than ours. His timing (rather than ours) will bring him greater glory.

HELP ME, LORD

Sometimes we are so sick or hurting so much that the only prayer we can say is, Help me, Lord. As God's child, you may be sure that prayer will be answered.

Charles H. Spurgeon, in his lovely devotional book *Morning and Evening*, talks of the Lord Jesus and his help for us.

Spurgeon says that the Lord Jesus might speak to us in this way:

> It is but a small thing for Me, thy God, to *help* thee. Consider what I have done already. What! not help thee? Why, I bought thee with My blood. What! not help thee? I have died for thee; and if I have done the greater, will I not do the less? *Help* thee!

It is the least thing I will ever do for thee; I *have* done more, and *will* do more. Before the world began I chose thee. I made the covenant for thee. I laid aside My glory and became a man for thee; I gave My life for thee; and if I did all this, I will surely help thee now.[2]

It may surprise us that one way God *helps* us is by making us aware of our total dependence upon him. Though this seems illogical, he can use our lives for his purposes only when we recognise that we must give ourselves entirely to him, so that he can be in complete control.

We often have the idea that the Lord wants us to work and strive, then, when we cannot quite manage by ourselves, call upon him to *help* us. God does not want to help us in this way. He wants our old *self* to step down and get out of the way so that he can do all of it *through* us.

Sometimes this truth becomes real to us when, facing the stark reality of our own infirmities, we meet circumstances totally beyond our control. Then we understand, as Paul did, that "My [Christ's] grace is sufficient for thee; for my strength is made perfect in weakness" (2 Cor. 12:9).

14

WHAT ABOUT MIRACLES?

The professing Church is caught up today in a tremendous emphasis placed on physical healing. On every hand we hear about miraculous healings through those who claim to have the "gift of healing". Nearly all of these people use the name of Jesus Christ.

Clearly, it is important for us to know and understand what the Bible says about healing, especially when we are confronted with a diagnosis of cancer.

Most groups that concentrate on bodily healing believe that all sickness is caused by Satan. Certainly, Satan is at the root of all sickness, since he is the one who tempted Eve to sin. In that sense, since he is behind the Fall of man, he is behind all sickness (see chapter seven).

But the Bible teaches various causes for specific sicknesses, some of which have nothing to do with Satan. If a person violates certain physical laws, he may get sick. Proper diet, exercise, rest, sanitation, and other things are necessary to maintain health. Violation of God's moral laws also may bring sickness. Scripture is clear that sometimes, but not always, God sends sickness to discipline his children (see 2 Sam. 12:15, 18; 2 Kings 15:5; and 1 Cor. 11:29–32). God also allows sickness for his glory and for our eternal good.

When sickness is brought on by Satan (and it sometimes

is), we must remember that God *has permitted it*. As Christians, nothing touches us except what God has allowed. This concept is clearly taught in the book of Job. Job was a God-fearing man who walked with the Lord. Satan wanted to show God that Job was faithful only because he had such a good life. God permitted Job to be tested—he lost his family, his wealth, his health. God used Job to demonstrate how faith can carry us through any trial. As for Satan, he could cause trouble only if God permitted. Even then, God set the limits.

This is not just an Old Testament concept. The apostle Paul had his "thorn in the flesh," a physical problem left unidentified, which he described as "the messenger of Satan to buffet me" (2 Cor. 12:7). Paul prayed for deliverance but found instead that God granted him grace to endure it.

Why did God allow Job and Paul to suffer? We cannot understand his ways completely, of course, but the fact that these two faithful servants also suffered is encouraging to us. It helps us to remember that even though we do not entirely understand, God does.

MEDICINE IS GOD'S GIFT

I believe medicine itself is one of God's wonderful gifts. God gave us intelligence and materials in nature to use. How, apart from the gift of God, would man have known to use roots, bark, oil, and wine for early medical cures?

Paul R. VanGorder, associate teacher of the American Radio Bible Class, says, "The Lord does not work miracles when human agencies can accomplish the required result."[1] It is foolish indeed for us to refuse to make use of the doctor's knowledge.

Though Jesus often healed in a miraculous, dramatic manner, he also approved the sensible use of medicine. VanGorder continues:

> Then, too, we saw medicine used when our Lord recounted the story of the Good Samaritan describing the condition of the man that had fallen among thieves who had beaten him, stripped him, and left him half dead. Jesus told us the Samaritan employed "oil and wine" in binding up the wounds. Both of these were used for healing in the time of Christ, and in fact they remain as two outstanding remedies today.[2]

WHAT ABOUT FAITH?

Those who promise healing usually insist that it is always God's will that a Christian be healed and that healing will take place *if the person has enough faith.*

The fact is that God does not always remove our difficult circumstances, no matter how much faith we have.

The writer of Hebrews tells of those faithful, godly persons who through faith, "conquered kingdoms, performed acts of righteousness, obtained promises, shut the mouths of lions, quenched the power of fire, escaped the edge of the sword, from weakness were made strong, became mighty in war, put foreign armies to flight. Women received back their dead by resurrection" (Heb. 11:33–35, NASB).

Up to this point, the account is very exciting, and it is clear that God performed many miracles. But the next portion is tremendously important and must not be overlooked. Sometimes we note the miracles that have happened in the past and assume that if we have enough faith the same miracles will surely occur in our lives.

Not all the heroes of the faith saw triumph over the physical circumstances of life. As we look at what their circumstances were, we know that these godly men and women suffered greatly in a physical sense:

> And others were tortured, not accepting their release, in order that they might obtain a better resurrection; and others experienced mockings and scourgings, yes, also chains and imprisonment. They were stoned, they were sawn in two, they were tempted, they were put to death with the sword; they went about in sheepskins, in goatskins; being destitute, afflicted, ill-treated (men of whom the world was not worthy), wandering in deserts and mountains and caves and holes in the ground. (Hebrews 11:35–38, NASB)

Anyone who reads the eleventh chapter of Hebrews is made aware of the tremendous sufferings, both physical and mental, that saints of former times endured. They showed their faith in the midst of terrible circumstances. Perhaps God wants us to do the same.

There are many instances in Scripture where removing difficult circumstances or physical infirmity was not part of God's perfect plan. Sometimes God healed and sometimes he did not. The same is true today. Sometimes God heals; sometimes he does not.

God uses illness in many ways, and it is shortsighted of us to think that he will always remove it from us (see chapter twelve for a discussion of reasons why God allows illness in our lives).

STRENGTH OF FAITH

The strength of our faith is not what counts either. The important thing is this: *in what* have we placed our faith?

Suppose two men are crossing a frozen river. The first man, fearful and shaking, timidly crawls out upon the ice, slowly and carefully moving inch by inch to the other side. This man has *little* faith. The other man is bold and confident. He moves across the ice with assurance and ease. He has *great* faith. As far as the journey is concerned, getting from one side to the other, the amount of faith is certainly not the issue.

Faith is involved in getting onto the ice in the first place, but what is important is the *object* of that faith. In this case the object of faith is the ice. If it is reliable, both men will get to their destination, whether they have little faith or much. The man with much faith will have a more pleasant journey, but both will eventually get to where they are going.

Likewise, the important thing is that we have placed our faith in Jesus Christ. Whether we are weak and scared or strong and bold is not the question. The important thing is the object of our faith—and he will not fail us.

Perhaps the man who was bold and confident on the ice had travelled over that frozen river before. The more we walk by faith, the more confidence we have.

I visited a cancer patient named Lois who was confined to her living-room couch. She was in physical distress because her cancer had spread from the original site of her breast to several vital organs and the bone. She had accepted Christ as Saviour but was still a baby Christian. Her daughter was very involved in a "healing" group and kept telling her mother that if she had "enough faith", she would be healed. From time to time the symptoms of the cancer would disappear, and she would think that her faith had been strong enough, and that God had rewarded her faith by healing her. Then, when she had a recurrence, she would say that her faith had "slipped". As time went on, and she became sicker, she became more and more guilt-ridden. Lois went to her grave believing that if she had had "enough faith", she would have been healed.

How cruel. Well-meaning and sincere Christians can be the cause of great grief.

Our God is great and powerful. He is no less mighty today than he was when he created the universe, or when he healed the sick in Galilee. He still has the power and authority to heal our physical bodies, and sometimes he does. But to promise a physical healing is to place my desire, based on limited human understanding, above his sovereignty.

From my own human point of view, I would love to be able to promise that God would heal your body. That would be so easy, and it would make you feel good. But God simply does not always work in the same way with each of his children. He may have far greater plans for his child in heaven than we can imagine here on earth. If we are disappointed that God has not healed, we must think that heaven is *inferior* to healing.

OTHER MIRACLE CURES

Besides miraculous healing, cancer patients are easy prey for those promising a cure for cancer with some new drug, treatment, or special diet.

Until medical science finally discovers the underlying causes of the various kinds of cancers—and permanent cures—quackery and fake cures will thrive. Sometimes people spend every penny they have on "cures" that do absolutely nothing to stop the cancer.

If you do decide to try some sort of treatment other than what your doctor has prescribed, tell him about it. It is important that you keep him informed.

BRINGING GLORY TO HIS NAME

Nell Collins says, "God leaves us here after we become his to bring glory to his name in special ways—ways that he chooses. Now one person might glorify him from a sickbed. Another person may bring glory to him while dying from cancer. Someone else may glorify him with extra good health or tremendous riches. The point is that we do not tell God which way *we* choose to glorify him. We accept his way, and then we begin to see how he can use for his glory something that seems like a tragedy to us."

15

IF I SHOULD DIE

Now I lay me down to sleep;
I pray thee, Lord, my soul to keep,
If I should die before I wake,
I pray thee, Lord, my soul to take.

Author Unknown

Many of us learned this little prayer as children. Over and over we repeated the verse, pounding into our subconscious the idea that we cannot know for sure that God will accept us when we die.

No wonder we are afraid of death.

To the cancer patient, the *process* of dying is often as frightening as death itself. But God does not leave us facing death with the kind of uncertainty expressed in this child's prayer. There is only one way to face death with confidence, and that is to believe God and what he has said in the Bible concerning it.

If you have been told that your cancer is terminal, you will probably be thinking more about death now than ever before.

DEATH AND DYING

Today there is tremendous interest in the subject of death and the process of dying. The mass media are bombarding the public with books and articles, while television interviewers probe the subject on talk shows. Colleges and universities all over the country are adding courses on dying. People talk more openly about death than ever before, thereby slowly erasing the taboos surrounding the topic.

People discuss death with doctors, nurses, psychiatrists, chaplains. Even some terminally ill people are being interviewed. But too often, even in our "enlightened" age, people face the end of their own lives with too little preparation, too little opportunity to talk openly, and too much pretending.

Generally, doctors have been taught to treat illness. They see death as the ultimate enemy and fight that enemy vigorously and courageously. To many doctors, however, death means failure, and some, sadly, find it difficult themselves to face the reality of death.

The patient is often the one who must set the tone as far as frankness is concerned. Tell your doctor you want to know everything, if you do. Tell the members of your family that you want to talk about dying, if you want the silence about it broken. You may need to be insistent, because they might be reluctant to discuss it. If *you* do not bring up the subject, however, they will probably be afraid to mention it. The more open and candid you are, the more honest they will be able to be. Great tension can be relieved by opening those lines of communication, and usually it will be up to the patient to do the opening.

The following are points that may help.

Preciousness of life. Dying is a part of life. Each of us is one day closer to his own death today than he was yesterday. Each day is very precious, and we should not waste our remaining time being miserable about the fact that this life must come to an end.

Living life to the full. No one knows how long he will live; no one can be sure what tomorrow will bring. But one does need to live each day to the full. If you are alive, God wants you to live for him. You still have work you can do for him, even if you are confined to bed. One lovely Christian woman could not get up from her bed, but she blessed hundreds of people by telephoning housebound invalids and writing cheerful notes of comfort to those in need. Some of the most effective and powerful prayer warriors are those people who are confined by illness or infirmity. Ask a pastor for a list of prayer requests. Pray specifically for the needs of missionaries and other workers. It will bring joy to your life to see how God will answer your prayers.

Hope for the grieving. It is not unusual or wrong to grieve about losing a loved one or one's own life. Jesus wept at the death of his friend Lazarus, and he grieved the night before his own crucifixion.

The family members grieve because they are losing a person they love. The dying person grieves because he is losing *everyone* he loves in this world. The Christian will grieve, but there is no need for us to sorrow as others who have no hope.

The believer, though he experiences grief, may cling to the wonderful promise of being reunited with his believing loved ones in heaven. This tremendous truth gives Christians hope, and it encourages them to speak of their faith to loved ones. Often a Christian who is dying will tell his pastor that he wants the message of salvation to be made very clear in his funeral service. He wants all loved ones who have yet to make a decision concerning Christ to know the *facts* upon which his faith was based.

Attitude of denial. Our society is saturated with impersonal death. We see thousands of fictitious people die on television, and sometimes, via the TV news, we see actual death occur. But when it comes to the reality of death in our own lives, death is largely denied. Medicine is seen as the saviour that will eventually conquer disease. Many healthcare professionals, unable to come to terms with their own mortality, commonly dodge discussions of impending death with the patient or his relatives.

Family relationships. Families who have close relationships before the onset of the serious illness seem to bear the distress of a terminal illness better than families who have not been as close. Families may withdraw from the patient. They seem unable to handle real communication because of their own fear and misery. Sometimes patients feel guilty because they have to rely on others for their needs. One person said she felt bad about "causing so much trouble for my family".

Families feel guilty about past failures and conflicts with the patient. This guilt may cloud the ability of the patient and family to communicate with each other freely. Reconciliation between loved ones can take place during this time, perhaps in a way not possible ordinarily. Do not hesitate to be the one to take those first steps toward mending broken relationships.

Loneliness of patient. Profound loneliness is often one of the most intense feelings of the dying patient. Studies have shown that nurses on the hospital ward tend to take twice as long to answer the buzzer of the dying patient, and doctors tend to make fewer and briefer calls on them, even though family doctors writing on the subject point out the great importance of frequent visits to both patient and family. Family members and friends often stay away because they do not know what to say.

Cicely Saunders, an authority on treatment of the terminally ill, reports: "A dying patient needs above all someone to listen and understand how he feels. Those who stay away from these patients because they feel they can bring nothing but their lack of understanding should realise that it is our desire to *try* to understand, and not our success in doing so, that eases the loneliness that is so hard to bear."[1]

Contribution of faith. It is interesting also that Saunders says patients with a strong religious faith were least anxious, while those with tepid faith were more anxious than those with none. She notes that there is a great difference between "intrinsic" and "extrinsic" religion. "Those who think of religion as a sort of insurance against trouble do not find such a belief sustaining in adversity, although they sometimes find a more mature faith when they are dying."[2]

FEAR OF PAIN

One of the strongest fears associated with the very word *cancer* is the fear that the disease will inevitably cause severe and untreatable pain.

Cicely Saunders states in *Nursing Times* that this is a misconception that can cause needless suffering.

"People live in fear", she says, "of the onset of pain, and, if it occurs, because it is thought to be inevitable, no complaint is made and no relief given. As a district nurse said sadly to us on a day visit, 'They don't know how much pain they are supposed to have.'"

She goes on to explain that 50 per cent of those persons who die from all forms of malignant disease should experience no pain at all. Another 10 per cent may be expected to have mild pain only. The more severe pain experienced by the remainder "can be abolished while the patient still remains alert, able to enjoy the company of those around him and often able to be up and about until near his death".[3]

She maintains that "successful treatment may call for much imagination and persistence."[4] If you are encountering severe pain that is not being controlled by your medication, you might suggest to your doctor that you would like to be seen by a doctor who specialises more in this area. Most doctors are glad to have a consultation and want very much for you to be as comfortable as possible.

The treatment for the more severe pain sometimes seen in terminally ill patients has been one of the major concerns of the hospice movement. The word *hospice* means "way station", and it is a facility, something between a hospital and a home, where terminally ill patients can receive the special care they need. The regular hospital routine, geared to saving lives and curing illness, in many cases has not met the needs of the terminally ill.

The hospice movement is simply an effort to meet the special needs of the dying, and it is really nothing new. Peoples in various cultures in both ancient and modern times have been concerned with the care of the dying. The problem has been that throughout most of this century, dying has seemed to be an affront to our great knowledge and technology. One writer says that there is a tendency in America to "regard death as a technical error and to write off the dying as if they were a business loss".[5]

The modern hospice movement began in England in response to the special needs of the dying and was brought about by an awareness that these needs were not being met. New hospices are being formed in cities all over this country. The hospice usually is a place where family members can be trained to care for the terminally ill at home. Most patients want to be at home with their families as much as possible. If, however, the patient needs more care than can be given at home, he can become an inpatient in the hospice.

Hospice personnel generally are dedicated to relieving pain and making patients feel cared for in a homey atmosphere, while still treating the disease as vigorously as possible. If you are interested in hospice care, call your local hospital. Personnel there should know where the nearest hospice facility is located.

WHAT IS DEATH?

Whether a person dies at home, in a hospital, nursing home, or hospice, he will face fears about the reality of his own death.

To the dying person, death is no longer the subject of abstract philosophical debate. It is real, it is imminent, and it is personal. God reveals to us truth about death, and a person who chooses to believe what God says about it is greatly comforted as his own death draws nearer.

The Bible speaks of two kinds of death: physical death is the separation of the soul from the body; spiritual death is the separation of the soul from God.

Our spiritual life begins with our union with Jesus Christ. When we receive him into our lives, we are "born again". This spiritual birth transfers us from the state of spiritual death into the state of spiritual life, and it is because of this fact that a Christian can go to sleep at night *knowing* (not hoping) that if he should die, he would immediately be with Christ (2 Cor. 5:8).

Man has been pondering death for ages. All kinds of ideas and theories have been proposed, based on man's speculations and fantasies. Archaeology has confirmed that people in every culture and civilisation have believed in a supernatural power, and that there is a universal belief that man's spirit does not die with the body. Hundreds of false theories about what happens after death have been popular from time to time, and many false theories are popular today.

How do we know these theories are false? God has given

us a divine yardstick by which we can evaluate any such theory. That yardstick is the Bible. If a theory goes against Scripture, it has to be false.

For example, here are some false theories believed by many people today.

No hereafter. This life is all we have, some say. Everything we shall ever have is right here on earth. This theory is popularly supported by beer commercials ("You only go around once") and familiar songs like "I'm gonna live 'til I die." Actually this theory is indirectly supported by the widely accepted evolutionary hypothesis, which leads to the conclusion that man is nothing more than a highly developed animal.

Annihilation of the wicked. The good live forever, it is said, but the wicked become nonexistent. This theory is popularly supported at funerals where emphasis is placed on how "good" the person was. "He was a good man," acquaintances say, implying that his goodness will earn him passage to heaven. The "bad" people, on the other hand, are simply blotted out. This false theory is called the "annihilation of the wicked".

Transmigration of the soul. The theory that the spirit of man goes on to live in another body is called "transmigration of the soul". This theory is often seen in the occult and Eastern religions, and is the basis for theories of reincarnation.

Universal salvation. Today the most popular theory of all is based on the fact of God's perfect love, and his perfect *justice* is forgotten. God is love, it is said, and a loving God wouldn't condemn anyone, would he? (It is precisely because God *is* love that he has provided a way, available to all, for us not to be condemned.)

These theories, interesting as they are, are false because they conflict with Scripture. They are dangerous, too, because they give people a false sense of security.

THE HUMAN SPIRIT IS ETERNAL

The Bible teaches that the human spirit does not die.

"And the Lord God formed man of the dust of the ground, and breathed into his nostrils the breath of life; and man became a living soul" (Gen. 2:7).

God created man perfect and eternal, and though sin destroyed man's perfection, his spirit remains eternal. Both believers and unbelievers have an eternally existing spirit.

Because of God's holiness, sinful man *cannot* spend eternity with him. To permit this would be totally inconsistent with God's holy nature. Therefore whoever sins is *alienated* from God during his physical life and separated from God throughout eternity. This state is called "spiritual death". This is the condition of the person without Christ.

According to notes in the *Scofield Reference Bible*, "Spiritual death is the state of the natural or unregenerate man as still in his sins." This person is "alienated from the life of God and destitute of the Spirit. Prolonged beyond the death of the body, spiritual death is a state of eternal separation from God in conscious suffering."[6]

Every one of us deserves to experience this eternal condemnation, because not one of us can meet God's standards of perfection. "For all have sinned, and come short of the glory of God" (Rom. 3:23).

THE GOOD NEWS

The word *gospel* means "good news".

The good news is that God loved us so much he sent his Son to die for us, to pay the penalty for our sins, so we could spend eternity with him. He did this at great cost to himself and offers everlasting life as a free gift to us.

Jesus was "raised again for our justification" (Rom. 4:25). Justification means the act of God whereby the sinner is declared righteous before him. We are not actually righteous. We are *declared* righteous. This declaration is based on the fact that Christ died for sin. It is not based on how much we *merit* this gift. A gift cannot be earned; it simply must be accepted. God declares us righteous because of what *Christ* did for us.

This makes possible going to sleep at night knowing that God accepts us. God accepts us because we accept his provision for us. If a person has trusted in Jesus Christ as his own Saviour, God himself comes to live in that believer in the person of the Holy Spirit. That is why Jesus could say to his disciples just before he ascended to heaven, "I am with you always" (Matt. 28:20; see Heb. 13:5, "I will never leave thee, nor forsake thee").

The apostle Paul knew that no matter what happened, he was assured of eternal life with God. As we face the future, whether it holds life or death, we can claim this promise: "For I am convinced that neither death, nor life, nor angels, nor principalities, nor things present, nor things to come, nor powers, nor height, nor depth, nor any other created thing, shall be able to separate us from the love of God, which is in Christ Jesus our Lord" (Rom. 8:38, 39, NASB).

Eternal life then is not merely promised for the future: it is the present possession of every believer. "He who believes in the Son *has* eternal life" (John 3:36, NASB, emphasis mine).

A NEW BODY

Believers may also be sure that someday our physical bodies will be transformed by the power of God into perfect, incorruptible bodies that will never get sick, never hurt, and never die. The ravages of cancer and the treatments for it can cause drastic, ugly, and even deforming changes in our bodies. The believer is given the wonderful promise that this situation is not permanent. We don't know how God will accomplish this great miracle, but we are assured in Scripture that he will. "We look for the Saviour, the Lord Jesus Christ: who shall change our vile body, that it may be fashioned like unto his glorious body" (Phil. 3:20, 21).

THE BLESSED HOPE

Christians are given yet another promise that is especially meaningful to those enduring trials. The Bible teaches that not all Christians will die physically. Those who are alive when the Lord comes for his church will be raptured, or translated, into his presence without dying. This event is commonly called "the rapture," and Christians of every generation have hoped that theirs would be the generation to experience this exciting happening.

In 1 Corinthians 15:51, 52, Paul explains the rapture: "We shall not all sleep [die], but we shall all be changed, in a moment, in the twinkling of an eye, at the last trump: for the trumpet shall sound, and the dead shall be raised incorruptible, and we shall be changed."

Paul is telling us here that those believers who have already died will be resurrected and their bodies supernaturally changed to be fit for heaven. Those believers who are alive at the time will not experience death, but their bodies will be instantaneously changed into perfect, incorruptible bodies.

"Then we which are alive and remain shall be caught up together with them in the clouds, to meet the Lord in the air:

and so shall we ever be with the Lord. Wherefore comfort one another with these words" (1 Thess. 4:17, 18).

It is, indeed, a blessed hope.

THE MOMENT OF DEATH

Though we have real confidence in our eternal life with Christ, and we can hope that the rapture will come soon, we still may have to face the moment of death, and we still may fear it.

Most of us have had little experience with the moment of death, because most people do not die at home anymore. People are usually taken to the hospital where the family is replaced by medical personnel and familiar surroundings replaced by a sterile environment. Perhaps this is progress, but I wonder if this, in a way, is a denial of death.

The moment of death may be quiet and peaceful, but often it is not. We have seen so many Hollywood deaths that we have come to expect meaningful "last words". Instead, there may be a convulsive struggle to live. Even for one with faith in Christ, the moment of death may be one final skirmish with the enemy. Usually, though, death comes quietly.

Albert Barnes, a beloved pastor and author of the last century, comments on the passage in Psalm 23, "Yea, though I walk through the valley of the shadow of death, I will fear no evil: for thou art with me."

The true believer has nothing to fear in the most gloomy scenes of life; he has nothing to fear in the valley of death; he has nothing to fear in the grave; he has nothing to fear in the world beyond. *For thou art with me.* Thou wilt be with me. Though invisible, thou wilt attend me. I shall not go alone; I shall not be alone. The psalmist felt assured that if God was with him he had nothing to dread there. God would be his companion, his guide. How applicable is this to death! The dying man *seems* to go into the valley alone. His friends accompany him as far as they can, and then they must give him the parting hand. They cheer him with their voice until he becomes deaf to all sounds; they cheer him with their looks until his eye becomes dim, and he can see no more; they cheer him with the fond embrace until he becomes insensible to every expression of earthly affection, and then he seems to be alone. But the dying believer is *not* alone. His Saviour God is with him in that valley, and will never leave him. On his arm he can lean, and by his presence he will be comforted, until he emerges from the gloom into the bright world beyond. All that is needful to dissipate the terrors of the valley of death is to be able to say, "thou art with me".[7]

Because the Spirit of the living God dwells within every believer, a Christian may know that he will never be alone. The God of the universe will be with him every moment, every step of the way. Before death, during death, after death—he will be there.

HEAVEN

What lies beyond the grave for the believer? A very real place. Not a figment of our imagination, not a dream, not a myth passed down from our more primitive ancestors.

Joseph Bayly, a man who has seen three of his sons die, writes about heaven in *The View from a Hearse*:

I cannot prove the existence of heaven.

I accept its reality by faith, on the authority of Jesus Christ: "In my Father's house are many mansions: if it were not so, I would have told you. I go to prepare a place for you."

For that matter, if I were a twin in the womb, I doubt that I could prove the existence of earth to my mate. He would probably object that the idea of an earth beyond the womb was ridiculous, that the womb was the only earth we'd ever know.

If I tried to explain that earthlings live in a greatly expanded environment and breathe air, he would only be more sceptical. After all, a foetus lives in water; who could imagine its being able to live in a universe of air? To him such a transition would seem impossible.

It would take birth to prove the earth's existence to a foetus. A little pain, a dark tunnel, a gasp of air—and then the wide world! Green grass, laps, lakes, the ocean, horses (could a foetus imagine a horse?), rainbows, walking, running, surfing, ice-skating. With enough room that you don't have to shove, and a universe beyond.[8]

Like the foetus, we cannot envisage what it will be like on the other side of the tunnel—in heaven.

But from God's Word we can know this much:

We will not be condemned. *John 5:24*

Heaven is a place of rest. *Revelation 14:13*

Heaven is a place without pain, weeping, or mourning. *Revelation 21:4*

Heaven is a place of total joy in the presence of the Lord. *Acts 2:28*

Though we will be changed, we will recognise our loved ones. *Matthew 17:3, 4; Peter recognised Moses and Elijah*

Heaven will be more beautiful than anything we can imagine. *Revelation 21–22*

We will be comfortable there, for it will be *home. John 14:2*

See you there, my friend!

Be Still, O My Soul

> O my soul, be not weary and troubled,
>   For God is still on the throne.
> Tho' the storms of adversity gather,
>   Remember, He strengthens His own.
> Tho' the lightning around you be flashing,
>   And the billowing waves o'er you roll,
> There is peace in the midst of the tempest;
>   There is peace, so be still, O my soul.

O my soul, be not sad or discouraged,
  For God is still on the throne.
Tho' the pathway of life may be rugged,
  Remember, you walk not alone.
The Saviour is with you each moment
  To lead you on mountain or knoll.
There is peace for the valley or summit;
  There is peace, so be still, O my soul.

O my soul, do not shrink from affliction,
  For God is still on the throne.
Remember the suffering on Calvary,
  An agony borne all alone.
Tho' the lengthening shadows of weakness
  Sweep the body in pain's dread control,
There is peace in the midnight of suffering;
  There is peace, so be still, O my soul.

O my soul, be thou quiet within me,
  For God is still on the throne.
Remember that nought should alarm you
  While He is protecting His own.
Tho' troubles like walls may surround you,
  And sorrows, like sea billows, roll,
There is peace midst the world's tribulation;
  There is peace, so be still, O my soul.

O my soul, do not weary of waiting,
  For God is still on the throne.
Remember, His promised appearing
  Will gladden the hearts of His own.
Tho' He linger a little while longer,
  His praises for men to extol,
There is peace, for His coming is nearer;
  There is peace, so be still, O my soul.

by Lillian Murr

APPENDIX

SITES OF CANCER

Just having solid information sometimes helps a person cope with cancer.

Cancer is classified on the basis of two primary factors: the type of tissue and the type of cell involved. In man, there are over 150 recognisable kinds of cancer. For convenience, cancers are usually grouped according to the part of the body in which the tumour first starts growing. Two other words are frequently used in cancer diagnosis: *carcinoma* and *sarcoma*. Carcinomas are cancers of epithelial tissues. These are tissues that cover a surface, line a cavity, or protect a surface. The external surfaces of the body (skin, breast) and internal surfaces (alimentary tract, organs such as liver, pancreas, intestines, prostate, thyroid) are all subject to carcinomas. Sarcomas are cancers arising in any connective tissue (muscles, cartilage, bone, etc.).

Leukaemias and lymphomas are generalised cancers which originate in either the bone marrow (leukaemias) or lymph nodes (lymphomas).

Usually, when a person dies from cancer, the malignant tumour itself is not the direct cause of death. Bowel obstruction, kidney failure, perforation, bleeding, and infections are some of the complications of malignancies that often bring about the death of the patient.

The following facts give us some idea of how cancer behaves in the most common sites of the disease.[1]

CANCER OF THE SKIN

Superficial skin cancer is the most common site of this disease, and it is the easiest to cure. Other than superficial skin cancer, the most common sites are the lung, the breast, and the colon and rectum.

Because superficial skin cancer is so visible, it is usually found early. Left untreated, however, this kind of cancer can also cause death.

Stanley Robbins in *Pathology* describes various types of skin cancer:

1. *Basal cell cancer*—This is the most curable of all cancers. It has a 98 per cent five-year survival rate.
2. *Epidermoid* or squamous cell cancer—This type is more serious than basal cell, because it has more tendency to spread to other parts of the body.[2]

Overexposure to the sun is the leading cause of skin cancer.

Malignant melanoma is not strictly "skin cancer", because it goes deeper than the skin and is more serious. It may have roots that penetrate deep into the body. It usually appears as a small, molelike growth that gets bigger.

Mycosis fungoides may involve other organs of the body. This is a form of lymphoma that affects the skin first. It appears as reddish, rounded tumours on the skin.[3]

CANCER OF THE LUNG

Lung cancer is the leading cause of cancer death in men. Scientists claim that this kind of cancer is largely preventable and that the primary cause of lung cancer is cigarette smoking.

Formerly lung cancer was rare in women, but the lung cancer death rate for women has increased 400 per cent since

1930. More women are dying from lung cancer because more women are starting to smoke at a younger age and are smoking more than ever before.

Two-thirds of the people who undergo surgery for lung cancer already have a metastatic tumour elsewhere in the body, so the survival rate is not as good as it could be if the disease were detected earlier.

CANCER OF THE BREAST

Breast cancer is the most common site of cancer in women. It is seen occasionally in men and rarely in children.

Most lumps are discovered by self-examination, and most are not malignant. Early detection is important, since it is vital to stop the growth before it spreads to another part of the body.

Surgery is the main treatment for breast cancer, sometimes in combination with chemotherapy and radiotherapy. The patient's ovaries may be removed, because some breast cancers are thought to be hormone-promoted.

Several different surgical procedures are used for breast cancer, and the most common ones are these:

1. *Extended radical mastectomy* or *supraradical mastectomy*—surgical removal of the entire breast, underlying chest muscles, the internal mammary chain of lymph nodes, and lymph nodes in the armpit.
2. *Modified radical mastectomy*—surgical removal of breast and lymph nodes in armpit.
3. *Simple* or *total mastectomy*—surgical removal of the breast, but none of the chest muscles or lymph nodes.
4. *Limited surgical procedures*—removal of the tumour mass and a varying amount of surrounding tissue and is accompanied by local radiotherapy. This type of procedure, sometimes called lumpectomy or tumourectomy, is controversial. It is increasingly used, but is reserved for extremely early breast cancer.

Most doctors recommend the radical or modified radical mastectomy, but many surgeons are now performing the initial surgery with techniques that will allow for reconstructive surgery later.

CANCER OF THE COLON AND RECTUM

The surgical treatment for this type of cancer is the removal of the bowel containing the tumour and adjoining tissue and the lymph nodes that drain the area. If extensive surgery of the rectum is necessary, a temporary or permanent opening in the abdominal wall can be used to eliminate waste. This is called a colostomy. After adjusting to the inconvenience of the colostomy bag, the patient can lead an otherwise normal, active life. Help and advice on the practical management of a colostomy can be obtained from the Colostomy Welfare Group, 38–9 Eccleston Square, London, SW1V 1PB.[4]

The cause of this kind of cancer is unknown, but many scientists believe that the Western diet—consisting of too much meat, not enough fibre, too much processing of foods—may have a great deal to do with it.

The following are some of the other common sites of cancer, listed alphabetically.

CANCER OF THE BLADDER

Bladder cancer is the most frequent malignancy of the urinary tract. The two main types of cancer of the bladder are papillary and transitional-cell carcinoma. The papillary type is more common and is the more easily cured. If detected early, there is a good possibility of complete recovery.

CANCER OF THE BONE

Bone cancer most often strikes children and young adults between the ages of ten and twenty. Relatively rare, it is usually diagnosed by biopsy, X ray, and isotope scanning.

Bone cancer originates in the skeletal tissues. Very often the bone is a site of metastasis from another place in the body, usually breast, kidney, thyroid, or prostate.

CANCER OF THE BRAIN

Cancers of the brain vary widely in their rate of growth, as well as their physical and chemical processes. Survival depends greatly upon which type of tumour is involved.

Brain tumours are almost always treated by surgery, often followed by radiotherapy. In the past, drugs have been less effective in treating cancer of the brain, because the protective membrane surrounding the brain could not be penetrated. New drugs have been developed, however, which are able to penetrate the "brain barrier". Researchers are also finding that using a combination of drugs can be effective.

Though seen most often in adults, brain cancer is the second most common cancer in children and has an especially high incidence in children aged five to nine.

CANCER OF THE LARYNX

Surviving cancer of the larynx, or voice box, depends almost entirely on how early it is discovered and treatment begun. The larynx is more accessible than some sites, and symptoms of this type of cancer (usually hoarseness) normally appear early, while the tumour is still small and localised. If the diagnosis is made early, when the cancer is limited to one vocal cord, the patient has a good chance of retaining the larynx.

Surgical removal of the larynx is necessary if the cancer has spread to other areas of the larynx and throat. Great strides have been made in rehabilitating laryngectomees, and across America clubs have been formed by laryngectomees interested in helping others learn oesophageal speech. This kind of speech is produced by expelling air from the oesophagus, and the great majority of laryngectomees have found it so successful that they have been able to return to full employment and lead otherwise normal lives.

LEUKAEMIA, LYMPHOMA, AND MULTIPLE MYELOMA

Leukaemia is cancer of the blood-forming tissues. It is not confined to a tumour in one place in the body. The leukaemia patient produces too many white cells. Normally the white blood cells help the body fight infection, but the leukaemic cells are undifferentiated cells and do not possess this capability. These abnormal cells invade all the organs of the body.

Cancer takes the lives of more children under fifteen than any other disease, and over half of these are leukaemia patients. Cancer is second only to accidents as a cause of death in children in the developed West.

The vast majority of children with leukaemia have *acute lymphocytic* (or *lymphoblastic*) *leukaemia* or *acute myeloblastic leukaemia*, and it is treated more successfully than other types, especially in younger school-age children.

The leukaemia patient has new hope because of the promising research of this area. New drugs are available that help him stay in a state of remission where the bone marrow can function normally again, and he can be free of symptoms. Bone marrow transplants are also being done with some degree of success, though this is still an experimental procedure and there are many unanswered questions.

More than 90 per cent of children with acute lymphocytic leukaemia will go into remission. Then the patient is put on a programme of drugs to keep him in remission. This is called "maintenance therapy" and usually is continued for three to five years. If relapse (or return of the leukaemia) should occur, the child will be put back on a programme to get him into remission again. Each time it gets harder to achieve remission.

A state of remission occurs when the leukaemia patient has no symptoms of the disease, and when the blood and bone marrow tests show no leukaemia cells. Remission is not the same thing as being cured; relapse can always occur, since a certain number of leukaemia cells, though unseen, are there. However, remissions are now lasting many years, and the patients can hope for the discovery of a permanent cure while in an extended state of remission. These leukaemic children in remission lead essentially normal lives. They look good; they feel good; they go to school.

Chronic myeloid leukaemia is an overproduction of all types of bone marrow cells, and it may be controlled for years.

Chronic lymphatic leukaemia may continue for twenty years or more.

The treatment for leukaemia in general is now predominantly by chemotherapy but may include radiotherapy, radioactive phosphorus, and other drugs. Sometimes blood transfusions, platelet transfusions, and antibiotics are prescribed.

Hodgkin's disease and *lymphoma* are solid tumours of the lymph glands and are closely related to leukaemia. Hodgkin's disease represents one of the major successes in the treatment of cancer.

Multiple myeloma is a tumour of the bone, which is

characterised by a proliferation of plasma cells and may show bone and soft tissue tumours.

CANCER OF THE MOUTH

Oral cancer occurs most frequently on the lip, then on the cheek and tongue. Other common sites of cancer of the mouth are the floor of the mouth, gums, palate, tonsils, lower jaw, and salivary glands.

The most common symptom is a sore that does not heal. Surgery and radiotherapy are used for treatment of cancer of the mouth, and highly skilled techniques of reconstructive and plastic surgery can be used to help restore areas affected by radical surgery.

Mouth cancer is strongly associated with cigarette smoking, excessive drinking of alcohol in combination with cigarettes, chewing tobacco, and using snuff. It appears to be even more strongly linked with pipe and cigar smoking. Chronic irritation from such things as jagged teeth and poorly fitting dentures can also cause mouth cancer.

CANCER OF THE PROSTATE

Prostate cancer rarely strikes men under forty, but after age fifty-five it is the third leading cause of cancer death in men.

The prostate is a gland in the male genital system. It is located just below the bladder. The symptoms for this kind of cancer usually involve urinary difficulty. If the growth is confined to the prostate alone, this gland is removed, and the chances for survival are excellent. If the symptoms become severe, and if there is evidence that the cancer is spreading, it is sometimes necessary to perform an orchiectomy (surgical removal of the testes) and administer hormone treatment.

CANCER OF THE STOMACH AND OESOPHAGUS

Stomach cancer is on the decline in this country, but the stomach is still a frequent site of the disease. Although scientists are not sure about the cause of stomach cancer, they tend to feel that diet is at least partially responsible.

Countries in which people consume great quantities of fish, such as Japan and Iceland, report a far higher stomach cancer incidence than Great Britain.

Oesophageal cancer is fairly uncommon in Great Britain. It is usually treated by surgery, particularly if the tumour is in the lower portion of the oesophagus. The portion of the oesophagus removed by surgery can be reconstructed from a section of the colon. The upper portion of the oesophagus can be treated by radiation. So far, anti-cancer drugs have not been found effective in treating oesophageal cancer.

CANCER OF THE TESTES

Although testicular cancer accounts for only about 1 per cent of all cancer in males, in men between the ages of twenty-nine and thirty-five it is the most common type of cancer. The prognosis after treatment for this type of cancer is excellent. The malignancy is nearly always confined to one testicle, and the remaining testicle usually retains complete fertility.

CANCER OF THE THYROID

Beginning in the 1920s and continuing for over twenty-five years, X rays were used to treat children and adolescents for such noncancerous conditions as ringworm, ear inflammations, inflammations of the sinuses, enlarged tonsils and adenoids, and acne. A link has been established between those X-ray treatments and an increased incidence in thyroid tumours in those people as adults.

Most of these thyroid tumours are benign, or noncancerous, and even when they are malignant, they are usually treated successfully.

CANCER OF THE UTERUS AND CERVIX

The first visible signs of cancer of the uterus are irregular bleeding or unusual vaginal discharge. Irregularities in the menstrual cycle, profuse periods, and the recurrence of a period after several months without periods are additional symptoms.

Uterine cancer may be treated by radiotherapy or surgery, or a combination of the two. Drugs, such as synthetic hormones, are also used in treating advanced cancer of the uterus. Surgery is performed to remove all of the cancerous tissue or the organ itself. If complete removal of the growth is not possible, surgery may still help to make the patient more comfortable and extend her life.

Cervical cancer responds extremely well to treatment and there is a recovery rate of over 90 per cent when caught at an early stage.

This look at some of the different types and locations of cancer has, of necessity, been brief. To obtain more detailed information about the type of cancer you are facing, contact BACUP (British Association of Cancer United Patients) at 121/123 Charterhouse Street, London, EC1M 6AA, who will be glad to send you information.[5]

NOTES

FOREWORD

1. Andrew Svvennsen 'Conquering Cancer' in the *Daily Telegraph* Sixth Form Essay Competition, 1986.

CHAPTER 2

1. Cancer Research Campaign data (1983).
   Office of Population, Census & Surveys' statistics 1983 (England and Wales), series MB1, no. 15.

CHAPTER 3

1. Elizabeth Ann Tierney, "Accepting Disfigurement When Death Is the Alternative," *American Journal of Nursing*, December 1975, p. 2149.
2. James Dobson, *Hide or Seek* (London, Hodder & Stoughton, 1982), p. 15.
3. Rene C. Mastrovito, "Cancer: Awareness and Denial," Memorial Sloan-Kettering Cancer Center, *Clinical Bulletin 4*, no. 4 (1974), p. 142.
4. Eileen Tiedt, "The Psychodynamic Process of the Oncological Experience," *Nursing Forum 14*, no. 3 (1975): p. 268.
5. Mastrovito, *op. cit.*, p. 142.
6. Maurice E. Wagner, *The Sensation of Being Somebody* (Grand Rapids: Zondervan, 1975), p. 146.
7. Mastrovito, *op. cit.*, p. 142.
8. Tiedt, *op. cit.*, pp. 264–265.
9. Mastrovito, *op. cit.*, p. 143.
10. Dobson, *op. cit.*, p. 135.

CHAPTER 4

1. Pat McGrady, *Science against Cancer* (New York: Public Affairs Pamphlets, 1962), p. 13.
2. Susan Golden, "Cancer Chemotherapy and Management of Patient Problems," *Nursing Forum 14*, no. 3 (1975), pp. 279–280.

CHAPTER 5

1. Megan Hudson, "She's 22 and Dealing with a Catastrophic Illness," *American Journal of Nursing 76*, no. 8 (August 1976), p. 1273.

CHAPTER 6

1. Mikie Sherman, *The Leukemic Child* (Washington, D.C.: U.S. Department of Health, Education, and Welfare, n.d.), p. 69.

CHAPTER 7

1. Lewis Sperry Chafer, *Major Bible Themes*, rev. ed. John F. Walvoord (Grand Rapids: Zondervan, 1975), pp. 42–43.
2. Merrill Unger, *Unger's Bible Dictionary* (Chicago: Moody, 1976), p. 668.

CHAPTER 8

1. "A Scientific Report on What Hope Does for Man," pub. New York State Heart Assembly, cited by S.I. McMillen in *None of These Diseases* (Westwood, N.J.: Revell, 1963), pp. 111–112.

CHAPTER 9

1. Darien B. Cooper, *You Can Be the Wife of a Happy Husband* (Wheaton, Ill.: Victor, 1974), p. 108.

2. Eileen Tiedt, "The Psychodynamic Process of the Oncological Experience," *Nursing Forum 14*, no. 3 (1975), p. 268.
3. Cooper, *op. cit.*, p. 106.
4. "Coping with Life's Strains,"; *U.S. News and World Report*, 1 May 1978, p. 82.
5. Tim LaHaye, *How to Win Over Depression* (Grand Rapids: Zondervan, 1974), pp. 53–54.
6. Armin Gesswein, *How to Overcome Discouragement* (Grand Rapids: Zondervan, 1965), p. 17.

CHAPTER 12

1. Maurice E. Wagner, *The Sensation of Being Somebody* (Grand Rapids: Zondervan, 1975), p. 146.
2. Hannah Whitall Smith, *The God of All Comfort* (Chicago: Moody, 1956), pp. 135–136.
3. James Dobson, *Hide or Seek* (London, Hodder & Stoughton, 1982), p. 36.
4. Henry R. Brandt, *The Struggle for Peace* (Wheaton, Ill.: Scripture Press, 1965), p. 5.

CHAPTER 13

1. Andrew Murray, cited in "The Christian and Prayer," in *Ten Basic Steps Toward Christian Maturity* (San Bernardino, Calif.: Campus Crusade, 1968), p. 4.
2. Charles H. Spurgeon, *Morning and Evening* (Grand Rapids: Zondervan, 1955), p. 32.

CHAPTER 14

1. Paul R. VanGorder, *The Bible and Healing* (Grand Rapids: Radio Bible Class, 1975), p. 10.
2. Ibid.

CHAPTER 15

1. Cicely Saunders, *The Management of Terminal Illness* (n.p.: Hospital Medicine Publications, n.d.), p. 23.

2. Ibid., p. 24.
3. Cicely Saunders, "Control of Pain in Terminal Cancer," *Nursing Times, Care of the Dying*, 2nd ed., 1976, p. 13.
4. Ibid.
5. Rose S. Le Roux, "Communicating with the Dying Person," *Nursing Forum 16*, no. 2 (1977), p. 145.
6. C.I. Scofield, ed., *The New Scofield Reference Bible* (New York: Oxford U., 1967), p. 1274.
7. Albert Barnes, *Notes Critical, Explanatory, and Practical on the Book of Psalms*, 3 vols. (Grand Rapids: Baker, 1977), 1:212.
8. Joseph Bayly, *The View from a Hearse* (Elgin, Ill.: Cook, 1969), p. 88.

APPENDIX

1. Most of the information in this section is from publications of the Public Health Service, National Institutes of Health, United States Department of Health, Education, and Welfare, Washington, D.C. 20402.
2. Stanley Robbins, *Pathology*, 3rd ed. (Philadelphia: Saunders, 1967), pp. 1298, 1301, 1309.
3. Ibid., p. 1353.
4. Another useful address is: Ileostomy Association, Central Office, Amblehurst House, Chobham, Woking, Surrey GU24 5PZ.
5. Cancerlink, 46 Pentonville Road, London N1 9HF, provides an information and support service for people who have cancer.